MIX
Papier aus verantwortungsvollen Quellen
Paper from responsible sources
FSC® C105338

Giorgi Gogichadze

Views and Suppositions about the pathogenesis of Cancer

disserta
Verlag

**Gogichadze, Giorgi: Views and Suppositions about the pathogenesis of Cancer.
Hamburg, disserta Verlag, 2016**

Buch-ISBN: 978-3-95935-192-8
PDF-eBook-ISBN: 978-3-95935-193-5
Druck/Herstellung: disserta Verlag, Hamburg, 2016
Covermotiv: © Uladzimir Bakunovich – Fotolia.com

Bibliografische Information der Deutschen Nationalbibliothek:
Die Deutsche Nationalbibliothek verzeichnet diese Publikation in der Deutschen Nationalbibliografie; detaillierte bibliografische Daten sind im Internet über http://dnb.d-nb.de abrufbar.

Das Werk einschließlich aller seiner Teile ist urheberrechtlich geschützt. Jede Verwertung außerhalb der Grenzen des Urheberrechtsgesetzes ist ohne Zustimmung des Verlages unzulässig und strafbar. Dies gilt insbesondere für Vervielfältigungen, Übersetzungen, Mikroverfilmungen und die Einspeicherung und Bearbeitung in elektronischen Systemen.

Die Wiedergabe von Gebrauchsnamen, Handelsnamen, Warenbezeichnungen usw. in diesem Werk berechtigt auch ohne besondere Kennzeichnung nicht zu der Annahme, dass solche Namen im Sinne der Warenzeichen- und Markenschutz-Gesetzgebung als frei zu betrachten wären und daher von jedermann benutzt werden dürften.

Die Informationen in diesem Werk wurden mit Sorgfalt erarbeitet. Dennoch können Fehler nicht vollständig ausgeschlossen werden und die Diplomica Verlag GmbH, die Autoren oder Übersetzer übernehmen keine juristische Verantwortung oder irgendeine Haftung für evtl. verbliebene fehlerhafte Angaben und deren Folgen.

Alle Rechte vorbehalten

© disserta Verlag, Imprint der Diplomica Verlag GmbH
Hermannstal 119k, 22119 Hamburg
http://www.disserta-verlag.de, Hamburg 2016
Printed in Germany

CONTENTS

PREFACE	7
1 PRIMARY TARGET FOR CARCINOGENS	12
2 DIFFERENT TYPES OF CYTOPATHOGENIC EFFECTS OF SOME VIRUSES	19
2.1 Fusogenic Effects of Moloney Virus on Lymphoid Type Cells	24
2.2 On the Common Genesis of Infectious and Oncogenic Viruses	28
3 FUSOGENIC EFFECTS OF WELL-KNOWN PHISICAL AND CHEMICAL CARCINOGENS	35
4 BIOTOXINS AND CARCINOGENESIS	40
4.1 Possible Correlation Between Bacterial Membranotoxins and Malignant Neoplasms	40
4.2 Cellular mechanism of cancer's induction by biotoxins of different origin on the example of hemolytic anemias	45
5 LOW PH, AS POSSIBLE REASON OF SPONTANEOUS MALIGNIZATION IN VITRO	50
6 REASON OF CANCER ARISING ON ALLOTRANSPLANTATIONS	52
6.1 Cancer cell formation by immune cytolysis	57
7 SOME "BIOLOGICAL NONSENSES" FROM THE POSITION OF THE KARYOGAMIC THEORY OF CARCINOGENESIS	60
7.1 Induction of malignant tumors by some fatty acids	60
7.2 Possible reason of induction of malignant tumors by some carbohydrates	64
7.3 Induction of malignant tumors by distilled water	66
7.4 Induction of malignant neoplasms by physiological solution (NaCL)	68
8 ONE AND THE SAME MECHANISM OF ACTION OF DIAMETRICALLY DIFFERENT CARCINOGENS	71
9 INITIATORS, PROMOTERS AND COMPLETE CARCINOGENS FROM STANDPOINT OF KARYOGAMIC THEORY	78
10 MOLECULAR GENETIC ASPECTS OF CARCINOGENESIS AT ITS DIFFERENT STEPS	84
10.1 Initiation	84
10.2 Promotion	86

10.3 Progression 89
    10.3.1 Invasion 89
    10.3.2 Metastasis 92

SUMMARY 97

PREFACE

Mankind, in particular its most intellectual stratum – scientists, can deservedly be proud of own progress in fighting some so far incurable infectious diseases, which used to do great harm to humans: smallpox has been liquidated, almost eliminated are Black Death, poliomyelitis; a great progress has been achieved in fighting tuberculosis, etc. At the same time, irrespective of great intellectual efforts and costs, some diseases, including primarily cancer, AIDS and others, are still beyond the human control.

Among the leading factors of science advance are hypotheses and theories, which originate at different stages of development of individual scientific disciplines.

A modern researcher of carcinogenesis is faced with the principal dilemma: he/she must either acknowledge that cancer is caused by completely different in nature agents and factors or try to create a theory, which will incorporate this array of conflicting facts and which make it possible to establish not only the role of a specific agent or factor in the development of cancer but also (most important) the possible mechanism of their action.

In the cancer research there were periods, when the research proceeded under dominance of researchers of different specialities. This rather complex problem was studied first by pathologists, then geneticists, immunologists and virologists. Naturally, such dominance was not of absolute nature. Lately the entire burden of this problem has been assumed by biochemists and molecular biologists. These very specialists are to reveal molecular processes in the cell genome anomaly, which cause the tumor process. From them we should expect the development of such methods which would contribute to curbing the spread of the disease or even to the process of its cure.

Tumors are widely spread in nature, the cancerous growth being one of the main causes of human mortality. Almost all types of multicellular organisms are practically prone to develop various forms of malignant tumors. Cancer (osteosarcomas) has been found in buried animals, namely in dinosaurs, which are known to exist long before the origin of man.

A rather alarming trend of tumor growth and "rejuvenation" has been observed lately. The spontaneous development of tumors is also frequently noted in laboratory animals, which makes it possible to study the neoplastic process experimentally.

The discovery of physical and chemical carcinogens has initiated a rather important stage of the theoretical oncology development. Almost all the phases of cancer formation and development are now observable. In general, the development of theoretical oncology is the most enigmatic page of the biological science history.

Experiments to study the cancer development in animals using different tissue irritators (acids, alkalis, etc.) have been running long since. In 1915, K. Yamagiwa and K. Ichikawa successfully induced the first experimental cancer by repeatedly painting coal tar into the skin of rabbit ears. Thereafter, rather potent carcinogenic hydrocarbons were isolated: dibenzantracene, benzpyrene, methylcholanthrene, urethane, etc.

A great number of factors causing tumor transformation undoubtedly essentially reduce a possibility of finding the general cause of cancer and of developing the etiotropic therapy.

Frequently, carcinogens of different nature tend to interact in a synergic action rather than exclude each other. All carcinogens have the like principal signs and properties, which, in certain cases, essentially coincide.

The circumstance that the tumor transformation of a normal cell is not a direct result of the action of a carcinogen, e.g. after irradiation, is seemingly indicative that the true cancer cell originates following a definite sequence of events taking place only at the cell and organoid levels, which requires certain time.

What is a cancer cell? Or what is its essence? At the current stage of development science has no answers to these questions. And by now, unless we understand the genuine nature of cancer cell, its essence, it would nor be real to think about the development of effective methods of treatment of this fatal disease.

It has been established that cancer cells gradually lose the structural and functional differentiation. At this stage, they become independent from the systems regulating the organism and corresponding tissues. One of the demonstrative examples of such autonomy is the tumor growth in a starving man, when normal tissues experience atrophy. A complex of cancer cells, as compared with the initial tissue, is of a more primitive structure, is anaplastic. For example, anaplastic cells of the mucosa sometimes do not mucify at all; the muscular tissue tumor loses compressibility and thus the main function of a living cell – specific synthesis of a respective tissue is altered. Some tumors start synthesis that is characteristic of the embryonic period.

In the opinion of the absolute majority of researchers working on the problems of carcinogenesis, the genetic apparatus of the target cell should be responsible for the conservation of a tumor cell from the normal cell. The role of non-DNA cellular elements in carcinogenesis has received little attention. A role for the plasmalemma in carcinogenesis has been proposed previously [1-4]. Out of the works dedicated to this subject (or the role of plasmalemma in forming a cancer cell) the most important, in our opinion, were the data of B. Israel and W. Schaeffer of 1988 [5]. It has been shown that fusion of cytoplasts from tumor cells with karyoplasts of normal cells resulted in a 97% incidence of tumors, while the opposite combination - fusion of normal cytoplasts and tumor karyoplasts yielded 0%

tumors in rats. At the same time, some scientists have proposed that genetic changes in carcinogenesis are on secondary place after unknown events on sub-cellular level [6]. Some scientists postulate the primary defect in carcinogenesis to be structural changes in the plasmalemma that result in loss of electron homeostasis [7].

However, the mechanism by which structural and biophysical changes of plasmalemma become persistent and heritable and their precise role in malignant transformation are unclear.

The essential positions of the karyogamic theories and malignant neoplasms genesis may be formulated in the following way: 1) malignant neoplasms may arise spontaneously, and also after the action on normal cells of various agents and factors of different nature. Primary target for carcinogens are determinants of cellular membranes, but not cell's DNA; 2) on the first stage of carcinogenesis (initiation) two normal somatic cells of one organ or tissue may create dikaryons - hetero- or homokaryons, but in some cases nonviable polykaryocytes. Presumably, during the perforation of cellular membranes induced by different carcinogenic and non-carcinogenic factors, the total charge of plasma membranes changes and the cells acquire the capability of closely approaching (adhesion), which frequently, especially upon coincidence of the perforated parts, may serve as a prerequisite to fusion process; 3) as a result of karyogamy, i.e. after synchronous mitosis or simple mechanical assembly of nuclei of hetero- or homokaryons, mononuclear hybrid precancerous cells develops, with tetraploid set of chromosomes on initial stage of hybridization. This is precancerous (initiated, immortal) cell, which exists in organism indefinitely long time; 4) influence of physical, chemical, and biological carcinogens on cells, is probably adequate. On the promotion stage, after the influence of complete (full) carcinogens or promoters on tissue, where precancerous synkaryons pre-exist, the chromosomal aberrations of different types and genes amplifications may arise in these cells. After the above-marked conversion on sub-cellular and molecular levels there may arise true cancer synkaryon – the malignant cell with the ability of uncontrolled proliferation. This cell represents clone, from which formation of malignant tumors substrate on early stage of carcinogenesis begins; 5) in a timorous synkaryon, in particular in its plasma membrane, most probably the antigenic mosaic of normal precursor cells is inherited, and due to this fact, such cells "escape" from the immune forces of the macro organism. And, actually, no specific tumor antigens, ferments, or the characteristic only to it different proteins, lipids, glycolipids or other chemical substances have been found in a cancer cell, which are not characteristic of normal cells at various stages of their life path; 6) in the process of tumor progression (concretely, invasion) after the segregation of some chromosomes, there may arise tumor cells with aneuploid or even hyperdiploid set of chromosomes. In extremely rare cases, tumor cells possess even diploid, hypodiploid or even hyperhaploid sets of chromosomes; 7) In the process of tumor progression (more specifically, invasion) segregation of some chromosomes in the tumor synkaryon, and also involvement last cells by means of fusion of considerably amount of other tumor cells and normal cells of different types and maturity take place. After this tumor cells with extreme polymorphism of karyotype and new abilities, arise. Evidently, the membrane potential of a cancer cell plasmalemma should be connected with the changes of physical and chemical nature occurring in the body, as well as with the metabolic activity of this type of cells proper. In the case of a relatively suppressed metabolism of cancer cells, the environmental pH increases. And in the case of high pH, a cancer cell may develop a high negative charge, which suppresses its adhesion with the tumor bulk and can lead to its detachment and migration in the macro organism (metastasis).

We have already published 4 books dedicated to the hybrid nature of cancer cell. One book is in Georgian (1993), the second - in Russian (1993), and in 2010 and 2013 monographs under our authorship were published in New York and Saarbrucken, dealing with the possible mechanism of malignant transformation of a normal cell [8,9]. They contain many facts in evidence of this idea, in terms of experimental and clinical medicine.

What did condition the idea of writing this monograph? And in what does it differ from its forerunners?

This the final attempt of writing a monograph dedicated to this subject (since all such earlier attempts, in the form of articles or monographs, with rare exceptions, have turned to be a "voice crying in the wilderness"). The main emphasis in this monograph, in contrast to the earlier monographs, is made on the first stage of carcinogenesis - namely on the initiation, which is discussed in detail (as far as possible!). The main steps of this stage, particularly the plasma membrane perforations and the resultant dramatic for a macro organism conditions, develop at the stages of cellular and sub-cellular levels. Moreover, as it has been found and as we will further see in all the chapters of the monograph, absolutely all carcinogenic agents, factors or effects are capable of forming in plasma membranes of target cells, the so-called pores, which in some cases may precondition the dramatic processes going on the cellular and sub-cellular levels.

Along with the experimental and clinical data, the opinions of theoretical nature, suggestions, etc., are given in this monograph to substantiate the karyogaimc theory of carcinogenesis.

In addition to the data evidencing the hybrid origin of a cancer cell, this work attempts to answer some important and still unanswered questions of modern oncology: 1.What is a cancer cell? 2.What is the essence of the common mechanism of action on the somatic cells of diametrically different carcinogens? In other words, how can so etiologically different factors, such as viruses, irradiation, chemical carcinogens, toxins, etc., cause the adequate carcinogenic changes in the target cell? 3.How the effects developed on the cell surface, in particular on the plasma membrane, cause hereditary changes in the cell genome? 4.Are the somatic aberrations the initial or secondary effects of carcinogenesis, etc.?

The book consists of 10 chapters with the seemingly radically different headings and contents, the unifying idea of which consists in the participation of diametrically different carcinogenic agents in the effects developed on the plasma membrane of somatic cells of different type, namely in perforations and follow-up somatic hybridization. Special attention is given to the evidence of the reality of initiation as the first stage of carcinogenesis, as well as the detailing of different steps of this stage.

The SUMMARY, given in the end of the book, is quintessence of the entire monograph being presented in the form of final conclusions.

The present monograph is not a manual to be read in succession, from the beginning to the end. Therefore, some main concepts, provisions are sometimes, although shortly but still, repeated in some chapters and sub-chapters. This will, to our mind, save the reader from unnecessary looking for a specific chapter or sub-chapter dealing with the specific subject.

REFERENCES

1. Tokuoka, S; Morioka, H. The membrane potential of the human cancer and related cells. *Gann*. 1957, 48:353.
2. Cone, D. Unified theory on the basic mechanism of normal mitotic control and oncogenesis. J. *Theor. Biol.* 1971, 30 :151-181..
3. Balitsky, K; Shuba, E. Resting potential of malignant tumor cells. *Acts Unio Intl. Contra Cancrum*. 1984, 20:1391.
4. Beech, J. A theory of carcinogenesis based on an analysis of the effects of carcinogens. *Med. Hypotheses*. 1987, 24:265-286.
5. Israel, B; Schaeffer, W. Cytoplasmic mediation of malignancy. *In Vitro Cell. Devel. Biol.* 1988, 24, 5 :487-490.
6. Prehn, R. Cancers beget mutations yarsus mutations beget cancers. *Cancer Res.* 1994, 54:5296-5300.
7. Stern, RG; Milestone, BN; Gatenby, RA. Carcinogenesis and the plasma membrane. *Med. Hypotheses.* 1999, 52, 5:367-372.
8. Gogichadze, GK; Gogichadze, TG. *Karyogamic theory of cancer cell formation from the view of the XXI century*. Nova Biomedical Books, New York. 2010.
9. Gogichadze, GK; Gogichadze, TG. *Somatic hybridization, as a primary reason of malignization*. Lambert Academic Publisher, Saarbrucken. 2013.

1 PRIMARY TARGET FOR CARCINOGENS

The study of a plasma membrane acquires a great importance in pathocytology, because it enables to obtain important data on the physiology and pathology of a cell. The critically important for a cell function – penetration, is closely associated with the plasma membrane. By means of this organoid a cell receives all necessary substances for extracting the final products of metabolism.

Any damage of a plasma membrane (e.g., perforation) by different effects leads to a direct contact of the damaged section of the cytoplasm with the environment, which might, in the case of large volume (size) of pores, cause the cell's disintegration.

The principal components of plasma membranes are lipids and proteins. Almost one-half of the mass of plasma membranes of mammalian cells is lipid. It is conventional to place the lipids in three different categories: phospholipids, neutral (uncharged) lipids (such as cholesterol, which is usually found in large amounts in plasma membranes, but not in intracellular membranes), and glycolipids. The lipids in membranes are arranged so as to accommodate their amphipathic character. They form a bilayer, who layers back to back, so that their hydrophilic heads constitute the top and bottom surfaces of the membrane and their hydrophobic tails are buried in the membrane interior.

Membrane proteins can be divided into two classes depending on their location with respect to the lipids of the membrane framework. 1. One class consists of those protein molecules that are associated only with the membrane surface. These proteins are located adjacent to either the outer or the inner surface of the membrane. 2. The second class is made up of proteins that actually penetrate the membrane surface. These proteins enter the lipid bilayer and sometimes extend all the way through it.

In the opinion of some scientists, especially of adherents of virus-genetic theory of carcinogenesis, it is hard to imagine that influence of cellular surface by different carcinogens may alter cells' genome; moreover, that inherited character of malignant transformation supposed exactly the cellular genome alteration. From the position of the karyogamic theory, the action of any carcinogen is not associated directly with gene apparatus of cells. Alteration of the cell's genome is induced indirectly; that is, after the somatic cells' fusion and arising of precancerous, tetraploid cell.

Thus, both viruses and other carcinogens of other nature contain in their primary target a plasmalemma of somatic cells rather than a genetic apparatus, as most suppose. Consequently, the primary and the principal target of different carcinogens (for example, viruses) is the plasma membrane of the cell. The irreversible damage of this organoid becomes the cause of the destruction of the cytoplasmic organoids and the cell as a whole. Some virus (and other carcinogens) through massive perforations of the plasmalemma, deranges homeostasis of the target cell, in particular, its metabolism, to which the cell respond with a whole series of second-order reactions. It is possible that upon massive attacks by the virus on the cell, formation of multiple disintegrations (perforations) in the plasma membrane, and penetration into the target cell, the same pathogen damages other membrane organoids of the cell as well (for example, lysosomes, mitochondria, endoplasmic reticulum, etc). To this should be ascribed the development of second-order morphological and functional changes in the target cell (for example, autolysis).

Presumably, any microtrauma of the cell surface provokes first of all injury, lysis definite part of plasma membranes. As it seems, upon massive infection of the plasma membrane and formation of pores of definite size, the cytoplasm gets in direct contact with the environment. And such type of a contact lead to the cytoplasm disintegration accompanied by edematization of its structures, enlargement of the sizes of the nuclei (disintegrative swelling), active movement of the ectoplasm as well as the cytoplasm, translocation of granules towards the nucleus zone. The cytoplasm consistently becomes diluted, indicative of which is the Brownian motion intensification. At the subsequent stages of cytopathology, when active destruction of the cellular organoid takes place, the damaged cell releases different intracellular components or their fragments: mitochondria, lysosomes, ribosomes, endoplasmic reticulum elements, intracellular vacuoles, lipid granules, disintegrated nucleus fragments, elements of the plasmalemma proper, essential for cell existence enzymes (e.g., protein kinases), etc., which catastrophically deranges its homeostasis. Thus, the carcinogenic and infectious processes, in spite of their principal difference (proliferation of target cells, in one case, and destruction - in the other), can be induced by the same agents (e.g., virus).

As regards the carcinogenic (initiated) action of some viruses, according to the karyogamic (hybridizationtheory, theory of "two synkaryons") of carcinogenesis, the primary and principal target of the virus (and other carcinogenic agents) is not the genetic apparatus of the somatic cell but the determinants localized on the cell's plasma membranes.

Thus, perforations of various volumes developed in target cell plasma membranes under the effect of some carcinogenic agents can become a direct cause of development of a wide range pathogenicity of these agents (infectious processes, teratogenic effects, carcinogenesis, immune deficiency, etc.). In more detailed see Chapter 2 about viruses). In other words: the biological sense of cancer (primary reason of malignization) consists in disintegration of somatic cells plasma membranes.

Adhesion is one of the most important general biological processes. Without this process the organogenesis and development of organisms in general would never happen. In embryonic tissues, especially at the early stages of their development, the intercellular connections are maintained by the adhesion. Besides, bacterial and viral infections are initiated by the adhesion (adsorption) process. The adhesion phenomenon consists of several stages, which leads to the attachment of microbial organisms to the epithelial cell surface. From one hand it is based on the non-specific physical-chemical mechanisms providing contact between the infecting agent and the target cell. From the other hand adhesion trend is defined by specific chemical groups represented by the ligandson the surface of the microorganism and receptors of the target cells corresponding to each other by the complementary principle. So there is no doubt that adhesion plays an important role in the organogenesis and infectology. Does it have any connection with the process of carcinogenesis?

As known, the superficial electric charge of most cells is negative. Factors, defining approachment of membranes, influence their adhesion, too. Before coming into contact, cells must overcome electrostatic repulsion of negatively charged surfaces of neighbouring cells. Some fusogenic agents, for example, PEG interact with glycoproteids and glycolipids, which are a part of the most superficial layers of cell membranes, and induce their alteration. The mechanism of action of PEG on cells consists of the absorption of molecules of this substance on the surfaces of cells and of the ability to bind ions of calcium. It is possible that molecules of PEG, when absorbed on the cell's surface, come into contact with cell's plasma membrane's outer layer _ glycocalix. Thus, the whole process of influence of fusogenic agents and factors, such as different viruses, electric impulses, chemical substances, etc., could be imagined in a following way: 1) contact on cells' surface; 2) modification or elimination of glycocalyx; 3) disorganization of cytoplasmic membranes (by means of perforation); 4) adhesion; 5) formation of common regions of cytoplasm between neighbouring cells; and 6) fusion.

As it is known, somatic cells never interact. There is always some type of space (intercellular space) between them which is roughly 100-200 A. As a result each cell maintains its autonomy as an independent unit. As it is thought the balance between the attraction and repulsion should be maintained at the 100-200 A interval. If for any reason the interval will become less than 10 A, formation of Ca bridges is starting leading to the long-term adhesion of the cell. Intercellular contacts are predominantly determined by two main factors: Van der Vaals (positive taxis) and electrostatic (negative taxis) forces contributing to the formation of membrane electric potential. Van der Vaals attraction forces develop trend towards approaching of two surfaces, while the electrostatic forces produce repulsion of the two surfaces. Presence of the intercellular space is a structural representation of the balance between the Van der Vaals and electrostatic forces [1,2]. It seems that pores in the plasma membrane of the somatic cells formed by the action of the different physical, chemical and biological agents, substantially decrease the negative charge of the plasma membrane. In different terms, this process (perforation) leads to the weaking of the elecrostatic forces and enhancement of the Van der Vaals forces helping somatic cells to overcome intercellular forces and enter into contact with each other. In the case of prolonged contact adhesion process will start to develop.

Malignancy should be ascribed to one of the rather wide-spread processes taking place in the organism daily and being, genetically inherited in a normal somatic cell. Among the processes in which the normal eukaryotic somatic cell-built programs participate during the body's vital activity, the following should be mentioned: mitosis, differentiation, interphase, phagocytosis, endomitosis, apoptosis, necrobiosis, adhesion, and, certainly fusing [3]. When speaking of the biological essence of fusing, its possibility to create polyploidy in somatic cells (like endomitosis) that intensifies resistance of a respective organ to negative environmental factors deserves mentioning. Regrettable, these necessary on the face for the organism processes (adhesion and fusion) are associated with the risks of malignant transformation of the fusion-developed binuclear and polyploidy cells.

By the karyogamic theory of carcinogenesis [4,5], initiated agents in the first instance interact with the cells' plasma membranes, inducing their perforations, contact, adhesion, fusion process and then cells' somatic hybridization (i.e. quantitative aberrations of chromosomes).

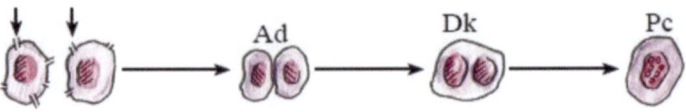

Fig. 1. Initiation

Abbreviations: ↓ - complete carcinogen or initiator;
= – perforation; Ad – adhesion; DK – dikaryon; Pc- precancerous cell.

Tumor cells may arise spontaneously, and also after the action on normal somatic cells of different factors of physical, chemical and biological nature. Initial target for carcinogens are determinants of cellular membranes, but not the cell's DNA. According to a work by Okada (1993), the fusion reaction does not require DNA, RNA or protein synthesis [6]. For development of malignant neoplasms, two normal somatic cells (even though one of them with a high potency to proliferation) and the factors inducing the process of somatic hybridization, i.e., complete (full) carcinogens or initiators are necessary.

In all probability, during the perforation of the cellular membrane, i.e., after the formation of pores (holes), induced by different carcinogenic (and noncarcinogenic) factors, the total charge of plasma membrane changes and the cells develop the ability to come closer to each other (adhesion), which frequently, especially upon coincidence of the perforated parts, will probably be the prerequisite to a fusion process [7-9]. Influence of physical, chemical and biological (viruses, biotoxins) agents on somatic cells probably are adequate.

Normal somatic cells (polypotent or commited cells sensitive to carcinogenic effects and capable of proliferation) form firstly a binuclear cells (dikaryons _ hetero- or homokaryons) and polykaryocytes by means of fusion with another cell of the same organism, in particular, with differentiated and non-differentiated cells of corresponding tissue or with cells capable to migrate (lymphocytes, macrophages, granulocytes of different maturity and so on). Thus, at this stage, together with multinuclear cellular structures, the binuclear cells, carriers of high carcinogenic potency, are formed. The majority of multinuclear cells probably do not proliferate.They are nonviable, nonfunctional formations and generally they break down and perish soon after.

At the initiated stage of its formation, tumorous synkaryons evidently possess a tetraploid set of chromosomes. Fusion immediately doubles the number of chromosomes, thereby decreasing the chances that the loss of some chromosomes will kill the hybrid (precancerous) cell. Thus, as a result of karyogamy, i.e., after synchronous mitosis or simple mechanical assembly of nuclei heterokaryons (or homokaryons), mononuclear hybrid precancerous cells develops, with tetraploid set of chromosomes in initial stage of hybridization. Received as a result of somatic hybridization, the hybrid synkaryon is an initiated, immortal, precancerous cell (synkaryon of stage I), which exists in macro organism indefinitely for a long time.

On the promotion stage, after the influence of complete (full) carcinogens or promoters on tissue, where precancerous synkaryons pre-exist, the chromosomal aberrations of different types and genes amplifications may arise in these cells. Following the segregation of some chromosomes, there may arise tumorous cells with hypotetraploid and hyperdiploid (on the whole, aneuploid) set of chromosomes. In extremely rare cases, tumorous cells possess even diploid, hypodiploid or even hyperhaploid sets of chromosomes. From the chromosomal aberrations, the most dangerous in carcinogenic respect are nonbalanced translocations, and also duplications, expressed in "complementation" of chromosomes' identical sites, having the same function. This event usually leads to genes' amplification, in consequence of which the expression of genes (oncogenes) responsible for the control under the cellular proliferation may ultimately originate. After this, the so-called "over-expressed gene" will arise. Following the above conversion on sub-cellular and molecular levels, there may arise a true tumorous synkaryon (so-called synkaryon of stage II), a malignant cell with the ability of uncontrolled proliferation. Synkaryon of stage II represents a clone, from which the formation of malignant tumors substrate at the early stage of carcinogenesis begins.

In some cases, carcinogenic agents (for example, viruses) induce twice or even triple cytopathogenic action on somatic cells: oncogenic (by formation of dikaryons), but in some cases, they induce arising of nonviable polykaryocytes and cytolysis in somatic cells, which may induce immune deficite of different degrees. Such different effects of carcinogens on cells depend on size of plasma membranes' pores. In the cases of comparatively big-sized pores, irreversible changes and cytolysis take place. Thus, practically all the agents and influences favoring cell's plasma membranes perforations and following of adhesion process, are regarded as the possible causes of the formation of tumor cell.

It could be concluded that physical, chemical, and biological carcinogens lead to similar results: to induction of cells malignization by means of adhesion, fusion and then somatic hybridization. Formed as a result of these processes, heterokaryons, homokaryons and synkaryons are to be considered as basis (substratum) of malignant growth.

CONCLUSION

Carcinogens contain in their primary target a plasmalemma of somatic cells rather than a genetic apparatus. Any microtrauma of the cell surface provokes first of all injury, lysis definite part of plasma membranes. Biological sense of cancer consists in disintegration of plasma membranes. Adhesion is one of the most important general biological processes. Before coming into contact, cells must overcome electrostatic repulsion of negative charged surfaces of neighbouring cells. Perforation leads to the weaking of the electrostatic forces and enhancement of the Van der Vaals forces, and the cells develop the ability to come closer to each other, which frequently, especially upon coincidence of the perforated parts, will probably by the prerequisite to a fusion process. Practically all the agents favoring cell's plasma membranes perforations and following of adhesion process are regarded as the possible causes of the formation of cancer cell.

REFERENCES

1. Policard, A; Bessis M. *Elements de pathologie cellulaire.* Masson et C ie, Editeurs. Paris, 1968.
2. Policard, A. *La surface cellulaire et son microenvironement.* Role dans les aggregations cellulaires. Masson et Cie, Editeurs. Paris, 1972.
3. Hallion, L. Sur la pathogenie du cancer; theorie karyogamique. *Press Med. Par,* 1907; XV: 10-11.
4. Gogichadze, GK; Misabishvili, EV; Gogichadze, TG. Tumor cells formation by normal somatic cells' fusion and cancer prevention prospects. *Medical Hypotheses.* 2006, 66, 1, 133-136.
5. Gogichadze, GK; Gogichadze, TG. *Karyogamic theory of cancer cell formation from the view of the XXI century.* Nova Biomedical Books, New York, 2010.
6. Okada, Y. Sendai-virus induced cell fusion. *Methods Enzymol.* 1993, 221, 18-41.
7. Arvinte, T; Cudd, A; Schulz, B. et al. Low-pH associated of proteins with the membranes of intact red blood cells. II. Studies of the mechanism. *Bioch. et Bioph. Acts.* 1989, 981, 61-68.
8. Siroki, J; Nebola, M; Pribyla, L. et al. Homokaryons from animal and plant cells generated by electrofusion. *Gen. Physiol. Biophys.* 1987, 6, 439-448.
9. Siroki, J; Cervenka J. Hybridization frequency of different mammalian cell types by electrofusion. *Gen. Physiol. Biophys.* 1990, 9, 489-499.

2 DIFFERENT TYPES OF CYTOPATHOGENIC EFFECTS OF SOME VIRUSES

The investigation of cytopathogenic action of viruses has long been in the center of attention of researchers. How and through what a mechanism does the so primitively organized on the face of it microorganism, such as a virus, manage to induce so wide a range of pathologies (infections, teratogenic effects, malignant tumors, immunodeficiency)?

It can hardly be said that virus cytopathology has been disregarded, especially as not only articles but also special monographs dedicated to the issue had been published long ago [1-3]. However, this quasi simple question is still awaiting a definite answer.

Already in the early 60s and 70s of the 20th century the action of a virus, namely the Sendai virus, on the surface of a cell (plasmalemma), was though to be the basis of induced fusogeny, although, no sufficient knowledge on the nature of this phenomenon was available by that time [4].

The interaction of a virus with the target cell is a complex and multistage process. As a result of such interaction, productive, integrative and abortive forms of virus infections are being developed. In the case of the productive form, the virus replication within the target-group's cytoplasm takes place, while in the case of the integrative form the virus nucleic acid is incorporated in the viral genome. The virus-cell interaction includes the following stages: 1) adhesion (adsorption); 2) penetration, or entry of the virus to the target cell; 3) transport of the virus in the cell; 4) deproteinization of the virion and release of the nucleic acid from the supercapsid and capsid; 5) eclipse phase; 6) composition of the virion; and 7) the virus egress/withdrawal from the cell through budding (complex viruses) or after cell destruction (simple viruses).

The virus penetration and budding stages have particularly attracted our attention, since it is exactly that time when the irreversible and reversible structural changes of the plasmalemma are being observed, which, in our opinion, can acquire a decisive importance in the possible development of some different, often diametrically opposite pathologies. How does the virus manage to penetrate the target cell? What is the specificity of its penetration to the cell? Is or not the so wide a range of pathologies induced thereby (infections, immunodeficiency, teratogenic effects, tumor growth) dependent on the specificity of the virus penetration to and withdrawal from the target cell?

There are 3 basic mechanisms of the virus penetration to the target cell: 1) receptor endocytosis - on the site of attachment to the receptor on the surface of plasmalemma (viropexis) invagination takes place, and then the vacuole (endosome) and the virus so get into the cytoplasm; 2) the virus disintegration and penetration of its nucleic acid into the cell at the site of adsorption (e.g., the so-called "microsyringe" (bacterial viruses) method); 3) the transmembrane (direct) penetration of the virus to the target cell caused by the plasmalemma perforation by virus enzyme. Massive penetration of the virus to the cell may trigger the cytocydic effects, or fusogenic effects upon small penetration of the virus. Seemingly, the direct cause of the cell plasmalemma disintegration (perforation) should be the specific activity of the enzymes of viral origin. Nonenveloped viruses deliver their genomes by a less obvious means and breach the hydrophobic barrier of the plasmalemma by pore formation.

The absolute majority of complex viruses leave the cell from the plasma membrane by the so-called budding. An exception are some complex viruses that are being budded from the karyolemma (herpesviruses) and the endoplasmic reticular structures (flaviviruses and coronaviruses), which, in the case of massive release from the cell, may also become a direct cause of disintegration of the target cell plasmalemma and further of the cell as a whole. Simple viruses, which are devoid of the supercapsid (picornaviruses, adenoviruses, etc.) lead to the cell destruction and are found thus in the intercellular spaces.

Some viruses (e.g., ortho- and paramyxoviruses) possess proteins: hemagglutinin and neuraminidase (the function of hemagglutinin consists in the attachment of the virus to receptors on the surface of the target cell, wherease neuraminidase decomposes the cellular neuraminic acid and facilitated release of the virus generation from the infected cell). At the same time, viruses of the paramyxoviruses family, with the exception of hemagglutinin and neuraminidase, have the so-called hemolytic (cytolytic) and symplast-forming factors. Supposedly, the hemolytic (cytolytic) factor (the same enzyme), will primarily affect the cell plasmalemma phospholipids. Seemingly, other viruses should also possess enzymes interacting with the plasmalemma receptors.

As it is known, the penetration to the target cell or budding of some viruses (retroviruses, togaviruses, paramyxoviruses, orthomyxoviruses, arenaviruses, poxviruses) results in the plasmalemma disintegration, triggering in the end perforations of different volume and amount. In other words, some viruses trigger massive perforations of the plasma membrane both "from without" (by penetration) as well as "from within" (by budding), during which the cytopathogenic effects of all types with completely different clinical manifestations are expected. At the same time, there are viruses (e.g., some simple viruses) that trigger perforations of the target cell plasma membrane only in the event of penetration.

As it seems, the intensity of virus infections and the virulent properties of the virus itself acquire a decisive importance in the development of all types of pathologies (e.g., infections, tumors, etc.), to be followed by the formation of pores of different volume and amount in the process of the target cell plasma membrane perforations in the process of penetration or budding.

Here should be mentioned the fact that the plasma membrane perforations can also be induced by the virus-associated immune cytolysis. For example, the humoral immune cytolysis has been described for the cells infected with the rubella, herpes simplex, lymphocytic choriomeningitis, tick-borne (wood-catter) encephalitis viruses, ortho- and paramyxoviruses, etc.

1. In the case of multiple penetration or budding, during formation of relatively large-volume (size) pores (approximately 8-10 to 100 nm) or upon their massive formation, rapid repair of the plasma membrane by the cell becomes impossible and the cell undergoes irreversible changes – destruction (cytolysis). Such an action, as it seems, should be characteristic of the highly virulent strain of some infectious viruses. In other words, viruses may cause infectious (and teratogenic) processes: a.by means of the sequential penetration and budding processes in the event of massive perforation of the plasma membrane (e.g., highly virulent influenza virus); b.by means of massive budding following receptor endocytosis (e.g., paramyxoviruses, togaviruses, retroviruses), and c.by means of the so-called post-receptor endocytosis "explosion" (simple viruses, e.g., reoviruses, adenoviruses, etc.), being accompanied with cell lysis. The clinical manifestation of such cytopathogenic effects can be infectious or teratogenic processes or both of them simultaneously.

2. In some cases, in the event of formation of relatively smaller pores, together with cytodestruction, viruses induce the formation of nonviable polykaryocytes (in the case of reversible changes of the plasmalemma) and cytolysis in somatic cells (in the case of irreversible changes of the plasmalemma), which may induce infectious processes, immunodeficiency of different degrees, or teratogenic effects (in the case of damage of the stem cells of any organ). The majority of multinuclear cells probably do not proliferate. They are nonviable, nonfunctional formations and generally they break down and perish soon after. Polykaryocytes are attending the carcinogenic processes of cellullar elements. In carcinogenesis they probably do not participate directly, but their presence in conforming tissues indicates to the probability of

creation of specific conditions for somatic cells' hybridization. Thus, actually all viruses that induce the formation of polykaryocytes (or symplasts) – paramyxoviruses, orthomyxoviruses, herpesviruses, retroviruses, adenoviruses, poxviruses, rhabdoviruses, hepadnaviruses, and many others [5-10], can be considered as suspected carcinogens (for they can, in parallel with the formation of polykaryocytes, form dikaryons with the high oncogenic potential). Generally, the cell-cell fusion mechanism of plasma membranes underlies the formation of polykaryocytes. As it seems, the polykaryocytes-forming virus that undoubtedly contains the plasma membrane-lysing enzyme (or enzymes) causes local damages to lipids layer of this organoid. The clinical manifestation of the formation of polykaryocytes in the macro organism's tissues can be an infectious process, immunodeficiency, or teratogeny.

3. In the case of the formation of pores of lesser size or amount, when reversible changes of the plasmalemma are taking place, the total charge of this organoid changes and the cells develop the ability to come closer to each other (adhesion), which frequently, especially upon coincidence of the perforated parts, will probably be the prerequisite to fusion process. Thus, at this stage, together with multinuclear cellular structures, the binuclear cells - carriers of high carcinogenic potency - are formed [11]. As a result of karyogamy, i.e. after synchronous mitosis or simple mechanical assembly of nuclei heterokaryons (or homokaryons) and then mononuclear hybrid precancerous cells develops, with tetraploid set of chromosomes in initial stage of hybridization. Received as a result of somatic hybridization, the hybrid synkaryon is an initiated, immortal, precancerous cell, which exists in macro organism indefinitely for a long time. From the formation of precancerous cell (synkaryon of I stage) to manifestation of tumor process or the formation of true tumorous cell (synkaryon of II stage), decades may pass. On the promotion stage, after the influence of complete (full) carcinogens or promoters on tissue, where precancerous synkaryons pre-exist, in these cells, the chromosomal aberrations of different types and genes amplifications may arise. Out of chromosomal aberrations, the most dangerous in carcinogenic respect are nonbalanced translocations, and also duplications, expressed in "complementation" of chromosomes' identical sites, having the same function. This event usually leads to genes' amplification, in the consequence of which expression of genes (oncogenes), responsible for the control under the cellular proliferation, ultimately may originate. After this, the so-called "overexpressed gene" arose. After the above-marked conversion on sub-cellular and molecular levels, a true tumorous synkaryon, malignant cell with the ability of uncontrolled proliferation may arise. This last cell represents a clone, from which formation of malignant tumors substrate at an early stage of carcinogenesis begins. Such an action can be characteristic of low-virulent infectious

viruses (e.g., influenza virus, some paramyxoviruses, retroviruses, etc.). Out of the numerous heterokaryons (or homokaryons) and hybrid cells (synkaryons) formed after the influence of viruses (and other carcinogenic agents), only a few precancerous cells can acquire the potency of unlimited proliferation [12]. In the overwhelming majority of cases, they seem to die in the phase of transformation into tumorous cells due to lethal mitosis. Specifically, because of the imbalance (instability) of karyotypes, they either never reach mitosis or are unable to complete it due to disturbance in spindle organization or chromosomes' motion. Therefore, true tumorous synkaryons are probably formed very rarely; their incidence being less than one in 10^6 [13].

Thus, in respect of oncology, dangerous are the low-virulent viruses which (1) penetrate the target cell through membranes, by perforations; (2) are released by budding; and/or (3) lead to cellular-immune or humoral-immune cytolysis.

Of special interest are the diametrically opposite cytopathogenic effects induced by the same virus and the resultant wide range of pathologies [14]. It is possible that the same virus could cause an infectious process and tumor growth, teratogenic effect, etc.? Or can we suppose that the diametrically opposite cytopathogenic and clinical effects are characteristic of only those viruses, which in the process of penetration or budding (or during the both processes) cause perforations of different volume of the plasma membrane of the target cell? Such viruses include: herpesviruses (infectious mononucleosis and Burkitt's lymphoma viruses), rubella (infectious process and teratogeny), influenza virus (infectious process and cancer), some adenoviruses serovars (infectious process and experimental cancer), etc. Especially as, according to some data [15-17], some infectious viruses of low virulence or low cytopathogenic action should possess fusogenic properties, or the carcinogenic potential. Such are vesicular stomatitis (rhabdovirus family), parotitis and rubella (paramyxoviruses family), herpesvirus (herpesviruses family), rubella (togaviruses family), and other viruses. The carcinogenic action of influenza virus has been experimentally established. Clinicians have repeatedly noted the association of the influenza infection and the recurrent viral pneumonia with the development of lung cancer, acute leukemia, and malignant tumors of other localization and histogenesis. In addition, in 70-80% of the anamnesis of the patients of the incological profile, influenza and parainfluenza disorders are being observed.

Thus, the infectious and carcinogenic processes, irrespective of a principal difference between them (the target cells destruction in one case and proliferation, in the other), in certain cases can be induced by the same virus. The seemingly typical oncoviruses, such as Rous sarcoma and polyoma viruses, can, in some cases, cause various non-tumor pathologies (inflammatory processes, hemorrhages, atrophy of internal organs, etc.), while infectious viruses may, under certain conditions, acquire the oncogenic potential. Therefore, the same virus in the case of different virulence and dosage can produce two or three types of diametrically opposite cytopathogenic effects.

2.1 Fusogenic Effects of Moloney Virus on Lymphoid Type Cells

According to the karyogamy (hybridization, two synkaryons) theory of tumor development, the cancer cell is a result of fusion of 2 somatic cells that may originate both by induction (carcinogenic agents and factors) and spontaneously. This certainly necessary and useful process for the cell and generally for the organism – fusogeny, which increases resistance of a respective organ (tissue) by way of polyploidy in response to different harmful effects, may develop first into a precancerous (hybrid, initiated, immortalized) and then into a true tumor cell. Carcinogens of different nature act apparently on normal somatic cels and by means of the common, universal mechanism (fusogeny) cause their tumor transformation [18].

Based on the principal postulates of the karyogamic theory, carcinogens, irrespective of their nature, should necessarily have fusogenic properties. At the phase I of the initiation, a hetero- or homokaryon with two haploid nuclei, the same dikaryon, is formed. Fusogeny should, supposedly, result from perforations of plasma membranes that can be caused by any carcino-genic agent, factor or effect. Because of definite size of perforations the negative total charge of the cell surface may change, enabling somatic cells first approach one another, enter into a close contact and cause thus adhesion, and then, in the case of coincidence of perforated sites of plasmalemma, fuse together. At the phase II of initiation stage, as a result of fusion of interfacial nuclei of dikaryons (as a result of their mechanical unification or synchronous mitosis), a uninucleate precancerous cell or a hybrid synkaryon (synkaryon of type I) is formed. Morphologically (phenotypically), precancerous cells resemble either the first or the second "precursor cell", or one of the initial cells, although differing from it genotypically. In some, as it seems, rare cases, based on the genetic law of intermediate inheritance, carcino-genic dikaryons may assume the characteristic of both partner cells so-called mosaic structure.

At the stage II of carcinogenesis, in particular upon promotion, first of all stimulation of the precancerous cells already existing in the tissues should occur, enabling the latter to return to the karyokynetic cycle and acquire a real possibility of conversion to a cancer cell. The transformation of a precancerous cell in a true cancer cell (synkaryon of type II) might have a molecular-sub-cellular basis, being expressed in structural aberrations of chromosomes (duplication, deletion, translocation, especially in an imbalanced translocation) and, finally, in the gene amplification.

In case of the karyogamic, the same "two synkaryon" theory reflects the real situation in oncology (at least partially!), it should be concluded that carcinogenesis is a polyetiological process and concurrently monopathogenic process. In other words, the causes of cancer are many agents, while the transformation of a normal somatic cell into the cancer one is caused by the common universal mechanism – fusogeny and the follow-up hybridization, although, as we will see further, fusogeny is fore-run by several phases provoking it.

Fusogeny of normal somatic cells may facilitate the genetic heterogeneity of precancerous cells, causing, in turn, the formation of tumor cells and further progress of the neoplastic process [19].

It is generally agreed that karyogamic theory of carcinogenesis is hardly subject to experimental corroborations. In our view, experimental material about this problem is available. (particularly, the data of Behringer [44] and our data, where we use so-call Moloney virus [45]). Given the notorious fact that the karyogamic theory is hardly liable to experimental confirmation, we believe it would be of interest to trace the early morphological changes caused in the lymphoid cells by the so-called Moloney sarcoma virus (one of the viruses causing experimental leukemia in mice). In case of fusogenic effects (formation of bi- and multinucleate cells) occurred in the lymphoid cells (especially as the Moloney virus reveals tropism in respect of this type of cells!), this fact would become one of the evidences in favor of the karyogamic theory. Furthermore, as known that the fusion of somatic cells has been found (admittedly, under experimental conditions) is caused by carcinogenic substances of chemical nature [20].

As is well known, different experimental mouse leukemia inducing viruses – C-type retroviruses: those of Gross, Graffi, Friend, Mazurenko, Moloney, Rauscher, etc. exist there. The lymphoid leukemia inducing Moloney virus was isolated from mouse sarcoma 37 in 1960 by the American researcher J. Moloney [21]. Said RNA genome virus belongs to a gammaretrovirus species of the retroviridae family. In BALB/c strain of mice, sharp activation of Moloney virus was achieved by gradual passing of the virus. Thus, for example, the leukemia latent development period was reduced from 6.4 to 2.5 months. The virus is devoid of strict specific differences. Thus, for example, the Spraque-Dawley strain rats as well as hamsters develop lymphoid leukemia. The diseased animals are noted for hepatosplenomegaly, mesenteric and peripheral lymphadenopathy and thymus hyperplasia.

The Moloney virus and the BALB/C strain 1.5-year aged, 20 gram 30 mice responsive thereto were used in our experiment. The virus concentration, which induces mouse leukemia in 100% cases, was administered intraperitoneally. To study the material (blood, bone marrow, lymph nodes), a light microscope and a transmission electron microscope were used. The material was microscoped in different time intervals (0.5 hr., 1-2-4-8-10-12 and 24 hrs). The same inbred mouse strain (BALB/c) was used as control without inoculation with the Moloney virus. The animals were killed in full compliance with euthanasia rules (inhalation narcosis).

A part of the infected mice (5 animals) was observed for approximately 3 months in order to identify the pathological process (lymphatic leukemia) in them.

On the basis of the carried out study it was found that already at the early stage of infection with Moloney virus complex perturbations of hemopoiesis took place, among which predominated the lymphoid tissue hyperplasia and the morphological changes developed in the lymphoid series cells.

The light microscope clearly showed intercommunication/contacts of cells, but not the fusion process. In general, the existence of contacts and furthermore fusogeny in the light microscope always gave rise to some doubts. Therefore, a detailed description of the latter type processes was carried out only using the electron microscope.

From the first hours of infection with the Moloney virus (2 hours and more), intercommunication, adhesion and fusion of the lymphoid cells were observed, being expressed in the formation of bi- and trinucleate cells. The fusogeny index (FI) of the fused, or bi- and trinucleate cells per 100 lymphocytes constituted 9-10 after 2 hours from the virus action, while their number though slowly but still increased and reached it maximum (15 cells) in the 8-hour material. Most fused cells had nuclei of the same type (characteristic only of lymphocytes), i.e. they represented homokaryons. The nuclei of the latter had different sizes and shapes, while their karyolemma (nuclear membrane) was frequently invaginated by different intensity. The different sizes of the cells bring out clearly the existence of fusogeny rather than endomitosis.

A rather small part of dikaryons and trikaryons was noted for nuclei of different type (e.g., lymphoid and granulocytic), or they correlated with heterokaryons. In case of both homo- and heterokaryons, irrespective of a comparatively significant magnification transmission of the electron microscope (15000 and over), no existence of the plasma membrane or its fragments between the cells was observed, which is another evidence of the fusogeny reality.

The fact that almost always only the differentiated lymphoid cells (and not the cells of other type) were present in the fusogeny process should be specially mentioned. This fact is another evidence of the lymphotropism of Moloney virus. It should be mentioned here that although very seldom but still there appeared heterokaryons, which is also evidence of the fact that the Moloney virus lymphotropism is not absolute.

Formation of the identified bi- or trinucleate lymphoid cells might take place through different processes, in particular by means of phagocytosis, endomitosis and fusogeny. In general, lymphocytes are known to have a weak capacity for phagocytosis. Therefore, it is unlikely that the identified cellular lump be formed at the participation of phagocytosis. As regards the process of endomitosis, the homokaryons so formed should, as a rule, possess nuclei of practically the same size and shape. Thus, significant alterations in sizes and shapes of the nuclei in the cellular formations (homokaryons) may be not ascribed to endomitosis.

Following the infection with the Moloney virus, perforations of the plasma membranes of the target cell (lymphoid cell) and the resulting fusogeny between the normal somatic cells may develop both "from without" – upon penetration of the virus in the cell, as well as "from within" – by the virus budding from the plasma membrane of the target cell.

In 2.5-3 months after inoculation with the Moloney virus, lympholeukemia was identified in 3 BALB/c strain mice, being further confirmed by a pathohistological analysis.

Thus, the precancerous (hybrid, initiated) cells having originated as a result of perforations and follow-up fusogeny of plasma membranes develop a better capacity of forming genetic alterations or of divergence. The further alterations of the genome, already at the stage of promotion, may be accompanied with the segregation and structural aberrations of chromosomes – non-balanced and reciprocal translocations, duplications, gene amplifications, etc. This, although seldom but still can induce the formation of tumor cells characteristic of lympholeukemia.

2.2 On the Common Genesis of Infectious and Oncogenic Viruses

As long as 1903, an opinion concerning the role of infectious viruses in causing malignant tumors was independently expressed by a French biologist A.Borrel and a Danish scientist F.Bosk.

An experimental verification of this excellent idea (virus theory of cancer etiology) was reported by two Danish scientists V.Ellermann and O.Bang [22]. They were the first to identify the virus etiology of chicken leukemia and some forms of tumors, by which a new promising direction in cancer research has been created. It should be also mentioned here that their report failed to attract proper attention of the then scientists, one of the probable reasons of which might have been disregard of leukemia as an oncological problem.

In 1911, an American scientist P. Rous showed that a transplantable, spontaneous spindle cell sarcoma derived from a Plymouth Rock chicken could be transmitted to healthy chickens using filtered cell-free tumor extracts [23]. Thereafter, in 1913 P.Rous with L.Lange described a filterable chicken angiosarcoma [24], whereas in 1914 with Murphy – the chicken osteosarcoma also transmittable by a filtrate [25].

Numerous attempts over the next decade to show a virus etiology for other cancers of mammals failed. An experimental research into oncogenic viruses started by an American scientist R.Shope in 1932 [26, 27] showed that wild cottontail rabbits contained a filterable agent from Papovaviridae.

In 1936, an American scientist J.Bittner discovered one more important oncovirus from the family Retroviridae [28]. He reported that certain mouse strains were highly prone to develop mammary tumors whereas other strains were resistant. Moreover, if cancer-resistant newborn mice suckled from a cancer-prone mother, they would show a high incidence of mammary tumors. Bittner showed that an infectious filterable agent, now called "mouse mammary tumor virus", was present in the milk of cancer-prone mice and transmitted the disease. Based on the above, it may be concluded that the oncogenic viruses may be only initiators of a carcinogenic process, rather than its promoters and, even more so, complete carcinogens.

One of the says in the development of experimental oncology has the discovery of an American scientists L.Gross, which led to the identification of the first mouse leukemia virus as a result of their radiation by X-rays in 1951 [29]. Thereafter, the similar mouse viruses were also isolated from the family of retroviruses through various methods and techniques by other scientists, such as Ch.Friend in 1956 [30], A.Graffi in 1957 [31], N.Mazurenko in the same year [32], J.Moloney in 1960 [33], F.Rausher in 1962 [34], etc.

The founder of the virus-genetic theory of tumor etiology L. Zilber [35] expressed an opinion on viruses (oncoviruses) running counter to the viral theory of carcinogenesis: 1) oncogenic viruses inherently transform normal cells into malignant ones; 2) viruses no longer have any role in further development of the already formed malignant cell; and 3) their action is principally different from the action of infectious viruses. In addition, according to Zilber, carcinogenesis is both a monoetiological (the virus being the single cause malignant transformation of normal cells) and a polypathogenic process (i.e. the malignant transformation pathogenesis is diverse).

Lately, both the virus and the virus-genetic theories have gradually lost their leading positions in oncology. Some scholars of authority (including some apologists of the virus-genetic theory) have opined that: 1) the virus may only be one of the carcinogens (together with chemical, physical and other carcinogens) rather than the single carcinogenic agent; and 2) the virus is more initiator of the carcinogenic process rather than being a complete carcinogen.

As the experimental and epidemiological studies show, certain infectious agents (viruses) of low cytopathogenic action also have, together with the oncogenic viruses, carcinogenic properties. These are: herpes, rubella, influenza, vesicular stomatitis, parotitis and other viruses [15-17].

In the works of Duran-Reynals (1943), the question was about the possible direct participation of the infectious viruses on the process of carcinogenesis [36].

Mazurenko (1957, 1962) successfully induced leukemia in mice by the inoculation of them to the influenza and cowpox viruses [32, 37]. It is also shown that cowpox virus, inoculated in small doses, induces neoplastic transformation in primary embryonic mice cultures. When inoculated subcutaneously in newborn mice, such transformed cells, on the site of inoculation, progressive malignant tumors appear. During the first hours of infecting the embryonic cells by the virus of vesicular stomatitis and cowpox, the appearance of multinuclear cells and symplastic structures was observed.

Moreover, the carcinogenic action of influenza virus has been experimentally proven. The fact that clinicians repeatedly mentioned an association of the influenza infection and the recurrent viral pneumonia with the development of acute leukemia, lung cancer and malignant tumors of other localization and histogenesis should also be underlined here. Furthermore, 75-80% of patients of the oncological profile are noted to develop influenzal and parainfluenzal diseases.

The above-mentioned experimental and clinical facts make it possible to conclude about the common genesis of infectious and oncogenic viruses.

By their structure and the development cycle taking place in a cell (morphogenesis), oncogenic viruses are identified with infectious viruses, which is indicative of their same genesis. They do not differ from one another by other characters – for example, by the proliferative and infectious reactions of the cells sensitive to them. The more so as there are such viruses (polyoma, Rouse, Moloney sarcoma virus), which, under certain conditions, cause the reactions of the both types, sometimes even concurrently. A clear-cut example of this is the Epstein-Barr virus (EBV), which causes infectious mononucleosis in one case and the development of a very aggressive so-called Burkitt's lymphoma in the other case.

At the same time, attention should be paid to the circumstance that while causing a malignant transformation of the target cell, the virus preserves its viability; the cell continues to synthesize acids and proteins, which is not characteristic of the virus and the target cell interrelation in the case of an infectious process.

Thus, the carcinogenic and infectious processes, irrespective of the principal differences between them (proliferation of the target cell in one case and destruction and lysis in the other case), can be induced by the same virus. The seemingly typical oncoviruses, such as the Rouse sarcoma and polyoma viruses, may become the causes of different non-malignant pathologies (hemorrhage, internal organs atrophy, inflammatory processes, etc.). The infectious viruses, on the contrary, can under certain conditions acquire the oncogenic potency.

The induction of the so radically different processes by the same virus may be dependent on the different pathogenic properties of the virus under different conditions (different virulence, dosage, the immune status of the organism, etc.).

The fact that some infectious viruses can cause the tumor growth process is not in the least indicative of the infectious etiology of cancer. In a carcinogenic process, beside the virus other factors should also be included in, so that their joint action could form a malignant cell [38]. Furthermore, it is the known in infectiology fact when an infectious disease, namely croupous pneumonia, is not contagious.

Thus, the distinction between the infectious viruses and oncogenic viruses is being gradually erased and acquires conditional character. In some cases, infectious virus is capable of modifying its pathogenic properties and serve as the initiator of the conversion of normal cells into malignant ones. In our opinion, the time when the distinction between the infectious and oncogenic viruses is completely erased and the double, sometimes triple cytopathogenic action (destruction, formation of dikaryons, or sometime polykaryocytes) of the virus on the target cell is finally acknowledged is not too far. It is possible that under certain conditions all the viruses (especially complex viruses) would develop an oncogenic potency.

We would like to deal briefly with the mechanisms taking place at the cellular and sub-cellular levels, through which the same virus may reveal both the infectious and oncogenic potency.

To explain the pathogeny of a viral carcinogenesis, we use the data of the karyogamic (hybridization) theory [39], under which any agent capable of fusogeny of somatic cells should be considered as the carrier of carcinogenic potency. The more so as many infectious viruses: Paramixoviruses (Sendai virus), Ortomixoviruses (influenza virus), Togaviruses (Sindbis virus, Semliki Forest virus, Rubella virus), Rhabdoviruses (vesicular stomatitis virus), also Retroviruses (HIV). As can be seen further, the fusogenic properties of HIV can serve as explanation of the facts of malignant tumors development in about 40% of the patients with AIDS.

Some experimental studies [40,41] have found that in the case of experimental mouse leukemia, from the first hours of infection with the virus, the somatic cells (the erythroid cells in the case of Friend's leukemia and the lymphoid cells in the case of Moloney leukemia) are noted for the fusogenic processes taking place in them.

From the karyogamic theory's positions, the primary target of the virus should be the determinants localized on the plasma membrane, rather than the somatic cells' genome. At the stage of initiation, in the case of massive perforations of the plasma membrane (the virus initiates perforations both "from without", or through the process of penetration into the cell, as well as "from within", or in the case of budding from the cell), the total negative charge of the plasma membranes reduces, the cells acquire the possibility of approaching, contacting each other with the follow-up adhesion. Not infrequently, especially upon coincidence of the perforated parts of plasma membranes, binucleate cells of high oncogenic potency – dikaryons (hetero- or homokaryons) or, in some cases, non-viable polykaryocytes may originate. At the same initiation stage, further development of dikaryons may take place: a uninucleate hybrid precancerous cell (synkaryon) may be formed as a result of karyogamy (synchronous mitosis or interphase nucelei mechanical fusion). At the formation moment, the precancerous cell has a set of tetraploid or hypotetraploid chromosomes, although further the chromosomes' segregation of various intensities may take place.

Seemingly, the decisive importance in the development of the virus-induced diametrically opposite processes (infection and tumor process) acquires the volume and number of the pores formed on the plasma membrane by the viruses. In the case of large-volume pores or their massive formation, the reparation of the plasma membrane by the cell becomes impossible and the cell undergoes destruction. Such an action should, seemingly, cause the infectious process. In the case of formation of the pores of relatively smaller volume, the phenomenon of fusogeny may take place to result in the development of a carcinogenic process with the formation of a precancerous (hybrid) cell at the initiation stage.

Thus, the same virus can, in the case of different virulence and dosage, trigger different (of two types) cytopathogenic effects cause, the clinical manifestation of which may be an infectious process, teratogeny, immune deficiency (in the case of cytodestruction) and a malignant process (in the case of cytoproliferation).

Given that a virus may in some cases induce the formation of precancerous rather than malignant cell, we can conclude that the virus is the initiator of a carcinogenic process rather than the complete carcinogen.

Further development of the virus-induced precancerous cell may proceed without any participation of the virus. Upon action of promoters or complete carcinogens on a carcinogenic cell, the cell might (although very seldom) be transformed into a genuine malignant cell, the basis of which are the molecular and sub-cellular changes (chromosomal aberrations – translocations, deletions, duplication, gene amplification).

CONCLUSION

The penetration to the target cell or budding of some viruses results in the plasmalemma disintegration, after perforations of different volume and amount. Some viruses trigger massive perforations of the plasma membrane both "from without" as well as "from within". At the same time, there are viruses that trigger perforations of the plasma membranes only in the event of penetration. The intensity of virus infections and the virulent properties of the virus itself, acquire a decisive importance in the development of all types of pathologies (e.g., infections, tumors, etc.). The plasma membrane perforations can also be induced by the virus-associated immune cytolysis. Thus, in respect of oncology, dangerous are the low-virulent viruses which penetrate the target cell through membranes, by perforations; are released by budding; lead to cellular-immune or humoral-immune cytolysis.

REFERENCES

1. Whitelock, O.St. *The cytopathology of virus infection.* New York Published by the Academy, 1959.
2. Luria, SE; Darnell, JE. *General Virology.* New York, London, Sydney, 1968.
3. Soloviov, VD; Khesin, YE; Bykovsky, AF. *Principles of viral cytopathology.* Meditsina, Moscow, 1979.
4. Harris, H. *Cell fusion.* Harvard Univ. Press, Cambridge, Mass, 1970.
5. Ichihashi, Y; Dales, S. Biogenesis of poxviruses: interrelationship between hemagglutinin production and polykaryocytosis. *Virology.* 1971, 46, 3, 533-544.
6. Chany-Fournier, F; Chany, C; Lafay, F. Mechanism of polykaryocyte induction by vesicular stomatitis virus in rat XC cells. *J. Gen. Virol.* 1977, 34, 305-314.
7. Kempf, C; Kohler, U; Michel, MR. et al. Semliki-forest virus induced polykaryocyte formation is an ATP-dependent event. *Arch. Virology.* 1987; 95; 1-2 :111-122.
8. Bentz, J. *Viral fusion mechanisms.* CRC-Press, 1993.
9. Shieh, MT; Spear, PG. Herpesvirus-induced cell fusion that is dependent on cell surface heparin sulfate or soluble heparin. *J. Virology.* 1994; 68 (2) :1224-1228.
10. Gao P; Zheng J. Oncogenic virus-mediated cell fusion: new insights into initiation and progression of oncogenic viruses-related cancers. *Cancer Lett.* 2011; 1 :303, 1-8.
11. Gogichadze, GK; Gogichadze, TG. *Karyogamic theory of cancer cell formation from the view of the XXI century.* Nova Biomedical Books, New York, 2010.
12. Gogichadze, GK. *Common characteristics of cancer cell and logical corroborations of its hybrid essence.* Advances in Genetic Research. Ed. K.Urbano. Nova Science Publishers, Inc. New York, 2011:161-178.
13. Little, JB. *Mechanisms of radiation transformation. Radiation carcinogenesis and DNA alterations.* Proc. NATO adv. Study Inst., Corfu, 1984, New York; London, 1986:155-162.
14. Gogichadze, GK. On the unified genesis of infectious and oncogenic viruses. *Georgian Medical Journal.* 2009; 2:18-22.
15. Vaananen, P; Kaarianen, L. Fusion and hemolysis of erythrocytes caused by three togaviruses, Semliki Forest, Sindbis and Rubella. *J. Gen. Virol.* 1980; 46:467-475.
16. Huang, RT; Rott, R; Klenk, HD. Influenza viruses cause hemolysis and fusion of cells. *Virology.* 1981; 110:243-247.
17. White, J; Metlin, K; Helenius, A. Cell fusion by Semliki Forest, influenza, and vesicular stomatitis viruses. *J. Cell Biol.* 1981; 89:674-679.
18. Gogichadze, GK; Gogichadze, TG; Kamkamidze, GK. Presumably common trigger mechanism of action of diametrically different carcinogens on target cells. *Cancer and Oncology Research.* 2013; 1 (2), 65-68.
19. Gogichadze, G; Misabishvili, E; Gogichadze, T. Tumor cells formation by normal somatic cells fusing and cancer prevention prospects. *Med. Hypotheses.* 2006, 66, 1, 133-136.

20. Gogichadze, GK; Dolidze, TG; Beniashvili, D. et al. Short-term bioassay for Confirmation of Carcinogenic Properties in Various Chemical Substances. *J. Conf. Int. Feder. Soc. Toxicol. Pathologists: "Current Methods for the Evaluation of Pathology in Toxicology", Nagoya, Japan,* 1992, 32.
21. Moloney, J. Properties of Leukemia Virus. *MCJ Monogr,* 1960, 4, 7-37.
22. Ellerman, V; Bang, O. Experimentalle leukaemia bei Hulnern. *Zentr. Bakt. Parasit. Abt.1, Orig.* 1908; 46:595-609.
23. Rous, P. A sarcoma of the fowl transmissible by an agent separable from the tumor cells. *J. Exper. Med.* 1911; 12:892-912.
24. Rous, P; Lange, LB. The characters of a third transplantable chicken tumour due to a filtrable cause: a sarcoma of intracanalicular pattern. *J.Exp. Med.* 1913; 18:651-657.
25. Rous, P; Murphy, JJ. On the causation by filtrable agents of three distinct chicken tumours. *J. Exp.Med,* 1914; 19:52-69.
26. Shope, RE. A filtrable virus causing a tumor-like condition in rabbits and its relationship to virus myxomatosum. *J. Exp. Med.* 1932; 56:803-822.
27. Shope, RE. Infectious papillomatosis of rabbits. *J. Exp. Med.* 1933; 58:607-616.
28. Bittner, JJ. Some possible effects of nursing on the mammary gland tumor incidence in mice. *Science.* 1936; 84:162-164.
29. Gross, L. Pathogenic properties and vertical transmission of the mouse leukemia agent. *Proc. Soc. Exp. Biol. Med.* 1951; 78:342-348.
30. Friend, Ch. The isolation of a virus causing a malignant disease of the hematopoetic system in adult Swiss mice. *Proc. Amer. Ass. Cancer Res.* 1956; 2:106.
31. Graffi, A. Chloroleukemia of mice. *Ann. New York Acad. Sci.* 1957: 68:540-588.
32. Mazurenko, NP. A possible blastomogenic action of infectious viruses. *Collection "Short Reports of Conference on Questions of Exper. and Clin. Oncology, Kiev,* 1957 :8.
33. Moloney, JB. Biological studies on a lymphoid leukemia virus extracted from sarcoma origin; an introductory investigation. *J. Nat. Cancer Inst.* 1960; 24:933-951.
34. Rauscher, FG. A virus-induced disease of mice characterised by erythrocytopoiesis and lymphoid leukemia. *J. Nat. Cancer Inst.* 1962; 29:515-543.
35. Zilber, LA. *Virus-genetic theory of tumor formation.* Moscow. 1968.
36. Duran-Reynals, F. The infection turkeys and guinea fowls by the Rous-sarcoma virus and the accompanying of the virus. *Cancer Res.* 1943; 3:569.
37. Mazurenko, NP. *Role of viruses in etiology of leukoses.* Kiev. 1962.
38. Andrews, CH. *The natural history of viruses.* Weidenfeld and Nicolson. 1967.
39. Hallion, L. Sur la pathogenie du cancer; theorie karyogamique. *Press Med.* 1907; XV:10-11.
40. Behringer, RR; LoCascio, NJ; Dewey, MJ. Erythroid cell fusion in the early phase of Friend virus leukemogenesis. *J.Nat.Cancer Inst.* 1987; 79:601-603.
41. Gogichadze, G; Beniashvili, D; Gogichadze, T. Fusogenic effects of lymphoid type cells at early stages of Moloney virus-induced lympholeukemia. *Exper. Clin. Med.* 2008; 5:9-13.

3 FUSOGENIC EFFECTS OF WELL-KNOWN PHISICAL AND CHEMICAL CARCINOGENS

1. The role of radiation in carcinogenesis does not give rise to any doubts. It known that not only the direct effect of radiation, but also the penetration of radioactive isotopes into the organism triggers the development of malignant cells. Together with the direct effect of the different kinds of radiation, the process of tumor formation may be also promoted by the penetration in the macro organism of radioactive isotopes. For example, radium (Ra. 226) penetrates into the bone, sediments in this organ and induces destruction of the bone tissue. This leads to development of incurable osteomyelitis. At the same time, there can originate malignant tumors, as well as hemoblastoses and osteosarcomas.

Transformation of normal cells into the tumor ones can also be promoted by the electromagnetic fields [1,2]. In the work of Hecht (1987), the increase of the cancer diseases among the children after the influence of weak electromagnetic fields, formed around the electric cables, lines and power stations was mentioned [3].

A new medical discipline – radiation hygiene has emerged and developed. It studies the ionizing radiation background formation and its doses, its effects on human health, also sets the sanitary rules and standards of radiation safety.

One of the famous representatives of natural radiation (together with ultraviolet rays) is the heavy gas, radon. Radon may induce lung cancer. Essential dose of radon were received by people in close buildings.

Thanks to the ozone screen, only small parts of ultraviolet rays (0.300-0.400 mkm) with high chemical activity reach the earth. Rays of this kind often induce basal-cellular and planus-cellular carcinomas. Melanomas, xeroderma pigmentosum (obligated precancerous state) use to particularly develop in fair men and in persons with very white skin.

The characteristic response of the macro organism to the radiation effect is massive destruction of lymphoid cells. This phenomenon is preceded by alterations in the permeability of the plasma membranes of somatic cells, followed by the DNA fragmentation, etc.

It is the established fact that in terms of oncology of special danger are low and medium rather than high radiation doses. Thus, a special carcinogenic danger represents weak (low-frequency) or middle doses of radiation. It is known that the majority of tumors are characterized by an increase in frequency of their formations with an increase of radiation dose to a definite level and reduction of frequency of tumors when exceeding this level of radiation. Probably, small doses of radiation can have initiating effects. Earlier, it was shown that the influence on precancerous skin (initiated by the chemical carcinogens) of necrotic dose of radiation reduced the output of malignant tumor. The other confirmation of this, so far, is the work of Berendsen (1987), which shows a tendency for increasing the risk of developing lung tumors after reducing the radiation dose [4].

Important changes have taken place in the radiobiological sphere lately. In particular, it has been found that in the case of low ionizing radiation doses the first target become the membrane components of cells. Although, it should be mentioned here that in the case of high radiation doses too, when the massive destruction of the target cell takes place, the primary target are still the plasma membranes.

As a whole number of experiments has shown, different kinds of radiation can trigger in the plasma membranes of somatic cells perforations of various sizes. For instance, high electro stimulation and prolonged impulses lead to partial increasing in the number of polynucleate cells, but further increase of stimulation induces cellular lysis. Under comparatively low doses of electro stimulation, dikaryons are observed most frequently, but polykaryocytes (multinuclear homokaryons) are revealed too [5,6]. After the application of break-down pulses binuclear cells were observed most frequently, but polykaryocytes also occurred. After cell contact fusion was induced by 1-10 pulses (1-5 kV. cm-1). A lower voltage (about 1 kV. cm-1) induced fusion of two or three cells, but at 5 kV.cm-1 cells also fused at various angles. The formation of polykaryocytes was also described at 6kV.cm-1 [7].

According to Kupers and Zimmerman (1983), the malignant transformation of normal cells leads to fusion after the influence on the organism of electromagnetic fields of the lighting discharge [8].

Ultrasonic homogenizers are a common tool for successful cell lysis.

Proceeding from the above, the version of the own electromagnetic radiation effect on the macro organisms at different range and power up to the development of malignant cells seems rather interesting and important. Such own electromagnetic radiation effects should be particularly frequent during stresses (especially in the case of distresses and eustresses).

Thus, the effect of the cells' fusion is a case of electric impulses possibly in base on electric puncture of cells' membranes.

2. The ability of the chemical substances to induce malignant neoplasms was first observed by English doctor Persival Pott (1775), who was the first to publish about the occupational cancer, resulting from the chronic exposure to a specific environmental agent, in particular, soot, chimney-sweep's cancer.

For the first time this idea was confirmed experimentally by Japanese scientists Yamagiwa and Ichikawa in 1914. Since then the method of artificial induction of cancer has been widely practiced in the laboratories of the world.

Hecker (1986) distinguished anthropogenic and natural chemical carcinogens and co-carcinogens [9]. Alongside the social factors (tobacco, alcohol) the most numerous groups are several industrial combinations and medical preparations. Now, there are known more than 1500 carcinogenic chemical substances and combinations. Their number constantly increases, because of the annual synthesis of a number of new substances.

The most well-known and drastic chemical carcinogens are polycyclic aromatic hydrocarbons (PAH), formed at incomplete combustion of any organic fuel _ methylcholanthrene, 3,4-benzpyrene, 9,10- dimethyl-1,2-benzantracene, etc. Aniline induces malignant neoplasms of the urinary bladder in workers of aniline industry. As appeared, malignant tumors developed as a result of long contact with the 2-naphtylamine, benzidin and other substances. Uretan induces lung tumors in mice. These tumors are benign and have a tendency to malignization. Numerous observations indicate development of cancer of the skin and the lungs in humans, and some malignant diseases of blood after the effect of arsenic and its combinations. Arsenic ingestion increases the risk of lung and kidney cancers.

Carcinogenic qualities of zinc, cobalt, nickel, beryllium, cadmium are proven by the experiments in laboratory animals, as well as by epidemiological researches [10]. Tamburro and Wadell have reported in 1987, about the induction of nasopharinx malignant tumors after the exposition to formaldehyde [11].

There also appeared the information about carcinogenicity of some pesticides. Non-Hodgkin's lymphoma and Kaposi's sarcoma has been associated with exposure to phenoxy herbicides [12]. These kinds of herbicides are known to be contaminated with dioxin.

It is interesting that dose-response relationship and oncogenic effect of low and middle doses in chemical carcinogenesis also take place. Thus, radiation of different kind and chemical carcinogenic hydrocarbons in great doses can induce intensive necrosis of tissue (cells), but more typical for them are "minimal effects".

The experiments conducted by us [13] have found that benzpyrene, dimethylhydrazine, 1,2-benzantracene and N-methyl-N'-nitro-N-nitrosoguanidine (NG) possessed the fusogenic properties of various intensity. The highest fusogenic activity was characteristic of dimethylhydrazine (the fusion effect – in 12-15% of cases). The obtained results enable to conclude that chemical carcinogens actively interact with the membrane components of a cell, causing the disorganization of this organoid or perforations, which finally leads to the fusogenic effect.

CONCLUSION

The characteristic response to the effects of radiation is the massive destruction of lymphoid cells. The phenomenon is preceded by the alterations in the permeability of plasma membranes of somatic cells, followed by the DNA fragmentation, etc. As has been found, different kinds of radiation can trigger in the plasma membranes of somatic cells perforations of various sizes. The experiments conducted by us have also revealed that different chemical carcinogens possessed fusogenic properties.

REFERENCES

1. Siroky, J; Nebola, M; Pribyla, L. et al. Homokaryons from animal and plant cells gene rated by electrofusion. *Gen. Physiol. Biophys.* 1987; 6:439-448.
2. Siroki, J; Cervenka, J. Hybridization frequency of different mammalian cell types by electrofusion. *Gen. Physiol. Biophys.* 1990; 9:489-499.
3. Hecht, F. Electricity blamed for childhood cancer.s. *New Sci.* 1987; 113:20.
4. Berendsen, JW. Effects of radiation on the reproductive capacity and proliferation of cells in relation to carcinogenesis. *Radiat. Carcinogenesis New York e.a.* 1987:85-105.
5. Zimmerman, U; Vienken, J. Electric field induced cell-to-cell fusion. *J.Membrane Biol.* 1982; 67:165-182.
6. Zimmerman, U; Vienken, J; Pilwat, G. Electric-field-induced fusion of cells. *Stud. Biophys.* 1982; 90:177-184.
7. Ahlbom, A; Feychting, M; Koskenvuo, M. et al. Electromagnetic fields and childhood cancer. *Lancet.* 1993; 342:1295-1296.
8. Kuppers, G; Zimmerman, U. Cell fusion by spark discharge and its relevance for evolutionary process. *Febs. Letter.* 1983; 164:323-329.
9. Hecker, E. Naturliche solitar-und kokarzinogene. *Schriftern. Chem. und Fortschr.* 1986; 2:24-32.

10. Tomatis, L. Identification of factors of oncologic risk and possibilities of cancer prophylactics. *Probl. Oncol.* 1987; 32:3-12.
11. Tamburro, CH; Waddell, WJ. Cancers the nasopharynx and oropharynx and formaldehyde exposure. *Natl. Cancer Inst.* 1987; 79:605.
12. Wesseling, C; Antich, D; Hogstedt, C. et al. Geographical differences of cancer incidence in Costa Rica in relation to environmental and occupational pesticide exposure. *Intern. J. Epidemiology.* 1999; 28:365-375.
13. Gogichadze, GK; Piriashvili, VA; Abesadze, AI. The action of some chemical carcinogens on nuclear erythrocytes. *Bull. Academy of Sciences of Georgia.* 1991; 141:397-399.

4 BIOTOXINS AND CARCINOGENESIS

The industrial human activity has long since acquired the global character. The contamination of natural components (air, water, soil, etc.) with radioactive isotopes and other toxic elements has taken place. The burning of buried fuel is a strong technogenic geochemical process. Upon incomplete firing of fuel and thermal processing of organic raw material a substantial quantity of toxic substances gets into the environment, as a result of which the possibility of human contact with different carcinogenic and mutagenic agents increases. Genetic, toxic, allergic and other kinds of diseases, the spread of which is closely associated with the environmental pollution have been identified.

According to the available experimental and epidemiological data, some biotoxins can trigger a malignant transformation of a normal cell. For example, the carcinogenic action of the mycotoxin – aflatoxin has been established. It is produced in great quantities by the the fungus *Aspergillus flavus*. Under conditions of high humidity and moderate temperature, this toxin is produced in great quantities. Aflatoxin induces malignant tumors in liver of animals and probably in man. Besides *Aspergillus flavus*, other mould fungi, which produce carcinogenic toxins (for instance, *Penicillium islandicum*, *Aspergillus ochraceus* and *Aspergillus parasiticus*) are known.

The study of biotoxins, namely of the membranotoxins of bacterial origin, is of special significance in this direction.

4.1 Possible Correlation Between Bacterial Membranotoxins and Malignant Neoplasms

Can bacteria cause cancer? Ever since 1890, when W. Russell described "a characteristic organism of cancer", there has been a small quantity of scientists who have claimed that bacteria cause cancer.

The idea that bacteria cause cancer was discarded a hundred years ago, and is still regarded as scientific heresy. Bacteria derived from cancer are generally considered as "laboratory contaminants". Thus, scientists have long suspected that cancer bacteria may be contaminants which infiltrate tissue cell culture, or invade cancer tissue after the disease has started as opposed to being a direct cause of cancer.

Over the past century hundreds of independent researchers have noted a link between bacteria and cancer, but their findings were treated as a scientific curiosity.

As the latest reasearch evidence, approximately 15-20% of cancers are caused by infectious agents _ viruses and bacteria. The infectious agents linked to cancer are not easily spread from person to person like the respiratory tract viruses (e.g., common cold virus).

In spite of the fact that the carcinogenic potential of some toxins (e.g., aflatoxin, dioxine, pesticides, etc.) has long been proved [1,2] the correlation between carcinogenesis and toxicology was finally established in the early 90s of the 20th century. Recently, a definite correlation between bacterial toxins and the possible development of cancer has also been found [3-7]. An overwhelming body of evidence has determined that relationships among certain bacteria and cancer exist.

It needs to be noted here that the cellular or molecular mechanisms of this phenomenon are still unknown. The bacterial mechanisms involved are as yet unclear. Therefore, many questions on theis sphere remain.

Some researchers think that the mechanism through which a cell manages to converse a normal cell to a tumor one is complex and should, as it seems, encompass a chronic inflammation, as well as a direct microbial effect on the target-cell physiology and the stem-cell homeostatic changes.

In this subchapter, we shall attempt to focus on exactly the presumptive cellular and subcellular mechanisms through which some toxins (in particular, baterial toxins) are likely to induce tumor conversion of a normal cell.

As it has been found, toxins of different origin, like different carcinogenic chemical substances, irradiation and viruses can, at different doses (virulence, in case of viruses), show *in vitro* diametrically opposite cytopathogenic effects (cytodestruction, fusogenicity), which will be correspondingly reflected in the clinical picture – beginning at general intoxication and ending with tumor growth. Aflatoxin, a mycotoxin of hepatotropic effect, has also been found to have the power of inducing diametrically opposite processes (e.g., necroses and tumors – hepatomas); nearly the same action is to be expected in the case of toxins released by other lower fungi (e.g., *Aspergillus fumigatus, Penicililum islandicum, Fusarium sporotrichiella,* etc.) and of the toxins of other origin. It has not been finally determined but gives a serious cause to expect the same ability and action on the part of some toxins of hemolytic action and generally of membranotoxins of different tropism. Furthermore, in the opinion of some researchers [8,9], some infectious viruses can also induce both the cytolytic (destructive) effects and fusion processes in somatic cells. Such ability of a double cytopathogenic action/effect is characteristic of orthomyxoviruses, paramyxviruses, rabdoviruses, togaviruses, herpesviruses, and HIV. Similar properties have been found in some oncogenic viruses (e.g., human T-cell leukemia virus).

Thus, completely different clinical presentations – infectious processes, intoxications, necroses, and tumors - correlate with the diametrically opposed cytopathogenic effects *in vitro* induced by toxins, viruses and other agents of different origin. Based on the above, infectious and carcinogenic processes can, irrespective of the principal difference between them (cytodestruction in one case and cytoproliferation in the other of target cells), be induced by the same agent: a bacterial membranotoxin, mycotoxin (e.g., aflatoxin), any infectious or oncogenic virus, etc.

Such double, diametrically opposed cytopathogenic processes developed in somatic cells by membranotoxins of different tropism (including hemolysins) must be apparently conditioned by: 1) different toxic doses; 2) different rigidity of plasma membranes of stem cells proper (e.g., erythrocytes, leucocytes, etc.), and, most important, 3) the so-called perforation degree, or pores of different size and number formed on the plasma membrane.

At the same time, based on the karyogamic theory of carcinogenesis, the initial target for any carcinogens are determinants of cellular membranes, whereas any agent or effect inducing fusogenicity shall be regarded as a potential carcinogen – or fusogenicity of somatic cells might lead to the formation of first a precancerous and then a tumor cell.

In order to prove the possible carcinogenic potential of membranotoxins of cytolytic effect and to demonstrate the presumptive mechanism of effect of these toxins on stem cells, we think it possible to cite as an example the acquired hemolytic anemia of different origin. As is well known, the induction of such a situation (or hemolytic anemia) occurs due to some exogenic hemolytic factors: organic (some snake, mushroom venoms, bacterial toxins) and inorganic hemolytic toxins (phenylhydrazin, arsenic, lead), infections, different drugs, radiation, burns, etc. In some cases, hemolytic anemia can be induced by antibodies targeted at own tissues (autoimmune hemolytic anemia). Antibodies (like cytotoxic cells) are known to induce damages (perforations) of different degrees of the plasma membrane of target cells. It has been established that 45-47% of patients with autoimmune anemia tend to develop malignant tumors. The analysis of patients with autoimmune hemolytic anemias showed chronic lymphatic leukemias, malignant lymphomas, multiple myelomas, ovarian cancers, etc. (in more detaied see suchapter 4b).

As rigidity of leucocytes' membranes is higher, it is possible that during destruction of erythrocytes (or immature cells of erythroid line) by hemolytic membranotoxins reversible damages of plasma membranes (pores of definite size and number) can be formed in leucocytes (or in other type of plasma membranes' cells of higher rigidity as compared with erythrocytes), which can promote the process of adhesion of somatic cells, leading further to the process of fusion in somatic cells and the formation of first precancerous and then cancer cells [10].

Also of importance we consider the circumstance that exotoxins of definite bacteria (e.g., toxins of *Clostridium perfringens* (0-perfringolysin), *Cl. septicum, Cl. histolyticum* and *Cl. novyi*, tetanolysin of *Cl. tetani*, toxins of *Cl. botulinum*, alpha-, beta-, and other toxins of *Staphylococcus aureus*, 0 and S streptolysins of *Streptococcus pyogenes*, pneumolysin of *Str. pneumonia*, I and II type hemolysins of *Pseudomonas aeruginosa*, cytotoxins of *Campylobacter* and *Helicobacter*, leucotoxin of *Pasteurella haemolytica*, 0-listeriolysin of *Listeria monocytogenes*, aerolysin of *Aeromonas hydrophila*, hemolysin of *Escherichia coli*, etc.) are really capable of rendering a strong membranotoxic (hemolytic, cytotoxic, neurotoxic, enterotoxic, etc.) effect on target cells of different types. One of the important causes of stomach cancer is long-term bacterial infection with *Helicobacter pylori*. Chronic ulcers as a result of the *Helicobacter pylori* greatly increase the risk for developing stomach cancer.

In addition, now available are the reports of other researchers on the pore-producing ability of some bacteria on the plasma membrane of target cells. For example, according to some authors [11,12], the *Staphylococcus aureus'* alpha toxin is the archetype of bacterial pore-forming toxins. According to Potez et al. [13], Annexin A6, is involved in the repair of plasmalemmal lesions induced by a bacterial pore-forming toxin, streptolysin 0. It has been also found that the perforation of the plasmalemma by membranotoxins (pore-forming toxins) causes an influx of Ca (2+) and an efflux of cytoplasmic proteins.

Membranotoxins affect primarily determinants of plasma membranes of cells that are tropic to them: they link to specific receptors of plasma membranes, provoke their lysis and, correspondingly, the development of perforations of different size and number in these organoids which can, in some cases, become a precondition for fusogenicity.

The possible carcinogenic potential of different gram-negative bacterial endotoxin should also be mentioned here. For example, supposedly, some strains of *E. coli* represent a risk factor for colon cancer development [6].

To all appearance, a decisive importance in the development of different type, often diametrically opposed pathologies (infections, tumors, etc.) acquires the so-called perforation degree, or the volume or quantity of pores formed in the target-cell plasma membrane by some toxins (and other agents). Based on the above, the following 3 options are considered below:

1. In the case of large-size pores (supposing approximately 8-10 nm and larger), or during intensive (multiple) intoxication, irreversible changes and cytolysis occur. In particular, high doses of a definite membranotoxin lead to the development of large-size pores: the cell fails to complete reparation processes and irreversible processes might be developed therein and result in cytodestruction (cytolysis). A clinical presentation of pathogenic effect can be an infectious process or a severe intoxication; while in the case of tropism to immunocompetent cells or stem cells, immune deficiencies and teratogenic effects may be induced, accordingly. Such an action should, seemingly, be characteristic of some bacterial exo- and endotoxins, as well as of the toxins of different origin.

2. In some cases, when pores of lesser volume or intoxication are developed, toxins induce simultaneous arising of nonviable polykaryocytes (in the case of reversible changes in the plasmalemma) or cytolysis in somatic calls (in the case of irreversible changes in the plasmalemma), and can provoke immune deficiency of different degrees (in the case of immunocompetent cells tropism) or teratogenic effects (in case a stem sell of any organ is damaged). Most multinuclear cells (polykaryocytes) formed as a result of fusion are not likely to proliferate. They are nonviable, nonfunctional formations that tend to quickly break down and perish.

3. In the case of formation of even lesser pores, when reversible changes of the plasmalemma occur (such an action is likely to be characteristic of both bacterial exo- and endotoxins and toxins of other origin), the total charge of this organoids changes and the cells develop an ability to come closer to each other (adhesion). This process (adhesion) frequently, especially on coincidence of the perforated parts, will likely become a prerequisite to fusion process [14,15]. Thus, at this stage, together with multinuclear cellular structures (polykaryocytes), the binuclear cells, carriers of high carcinogenic potency, are formed. As a result of karyogamy, i.e. after synchronous mitosis or simple mechanical assembly of nuclei heterokaryons (or homokaryons), mononuclear hybrid precancerous cells develop with a tetraploid set of chromosomes in the initial stage of hybridiza-

tion. Toxins (and other pathogenic agents, e.g., viruses) strongly stimulate the occurrence of chromosomal abnormalities in these cells. The hybrid synkaryon produced as a result of somatic hybridization is an initiated, immortal, precancerous cell which can exist in a macro organism indefinitely for a long time. From the formation of the precancerous cell (I stage synkaryon) to the manifestation of a tumor process or the formation of a true cancer cell (II stage synkaryon), decades may pass. On the promotion stage, after the effect of complete (full) carcinogens or promoters or the same toxin on tissue, where precancerous cells pre-exist, the chromosomal aberrations of different types and gene amplifications may arise in these cells. From among the chromosomal aberrations, the most dangerous in the carcinogenic respect are imbalanced translocations, also duplications being expressed as "complementation" of chromosomes' identical sites and having the same function. This event usually leads to the amplification of genes, in the consequence of which an expression of genes (oncogenes) responsible for control under the cellular proliferation will ultimately originate. After this, so-called "over-expressed gene" arose. After above-marked conversion on sub-cellular and molecular levels, there may arise true tumorous synkaryon, malignant cell with the ability of uncontrolled proliferation. This last cell represents a clone, from which the formation of malignant tumor substrate at the early stage of carcinogenesis commences.

Thus, some bacterial membranotoxins of different tropism are capable, as a result of damages of the plasma membrane of the target cell of various degrees (perforation, lysis), of inducing both infectious processes as well as the formation of first precancerous and then cancer cells.

4.2 Cellular mechanism of cancer's induction by biotoxins of different origin on the example of hemolytic anemias

There are hemolytic anemias of different origin. For instance, these states may be induced by means of some exogenic hemolytic factors: by different organic and unorganic hemolytic toxins (phosphorus, phenylhydrazin, saponins, arsenicum, lead and biotoxins – snake venom, mushroom poisons, mycotoxins, etc.), some medical preparations, radiations, some infectious agents and haevy burns. Besides, in some cases, hemolytic anemias are induced by antibodies against own tissues (autoimmune hemolytic anaemia). Reason of immunization of autoimmune hemolytic anemias may be infection diseases (grippe, malaria, acute anaerobic or streptococcal sepsis, pneumonias, i.e. viruses, bacteria, mycoplasma and so on) and some other physical and chemical factors and influences.

A strong relationship exists between autoimmunity and B-cell oncogenesis. According to clinical studies malignant tumors in autoimmune hemolytic anemias appear in 45-47%. Observation of a large body of literature, as well as our experience permit to suggest that quite frequently tumor cells in autoimmune hemolytic anemias have lymphoid and macrophagal nature. The analysis of 234 patients with autoimmune hemolytic anemias showed chronic lympholeukemias, malignant lymphomas, multiple myelomas and so on [16]. The analysis of 168 patients with hemolytic anemias showed approximately similar results [17].

At the same time in the opinion of some scientists, some toxins, even different infectious viruses (for instance, viruses of grippe, rubella and HIV) and carcinogenic agents may induce both fusion process and cytolytic (destructive) effects in somatic cells. Such different effects of these agents on somatic cells possibly depend on the size of plasma membranes' pores induced by them. In the case of large pores irreversible changes and cytolysis take place. For instance, high doses of carcinogenic agents lead to partial increasing of quantity of giant polynuclear cells, but further increase of this dose induces massive cellular lysis. In a case of these agents tropism to immunocompetent cells, immune deficite of different degree may be induced. In low doses of carcinogenic agents, dikaryons are observed most frequently.

In the present subchapter we have the aim to explain the cellular mechanism of development of malignant tumors in hemolytic anemias, in particular, malignant lymphoid and macrophagal tumors.

As rigidity of leucocytes' membranes is higher, it is possible that during destruction of erythrocytes (or immature cells of this line) by some agents (carcinogens, some toxins, infectious viruses, antibiotics, antibodies, etc.), in leucocytes damages of plasma membranes and pores of definite size, which may promote process of fusion of somatic cells, may be formed. Larger perforations induce considerable destruction of cell membranes and following cytolysis together with the perishing of these cells.

Thus, in hemolytic anemias of different genesis side by side with hemolysis, process of somatic cells fusion may take place. For instance, after bite of snake with hemolytic action of venom (*Vipera lebetina, Vipera Russellii*, etc.) together with massive destruction of erythrocytes (hemolysis), there may be induced a fusion process of other cellular types with more rigid plasma membranes (for instance, leucocytes of different maturity, and probably of cells of other type), with possible development of precancerous, and then true malignant cell. Approximately similar action one may expect from fungus toxins (*Aspergillus flavus, Penicil-*

lium islandicum, Aspergillus ochraceus, etc.). For instance, toxin of *Aspergillus flavus* – aflatoxin, together with heavy toxic action, induces malignant tumors (hepatomas) of the liver.

We have conducted a special experiment for the determination of cytopathogenic action of viper's (*Vipera lebetina*) venom in short-term cellular culture (avian blood). There are some assumptions about the association of *Vipera lebetina* bites with the development of cancer of different localization and histogenesis.

The definition of fusogenic concentration of the Vipera lebetina venom was done empirically - at the first step the lethal (maximal dose) concentration of the venom was identified which has an ability to induce hemolysis in 100% of erythrocytes already after 0,5 hour of exposition. At the next step the venom concentration was decreased gradually and in parallel cytopathogenic changes in erythrocytes and leucocytes was investigated. It was shown that 100% hemolytic action was induced by the biotoxin's concentration equal to 20 mkg/ml. This concentration induced hemolytic effect at 0,5 hour after the exposition.

Lower doses of *Vipera lebetina* venom (10 mkg/ml) after a 2-hour exposition to blood cells induce a weak fusogenic effect. The number of fused cells (double or in more rare cases triple-nuclear cells) per 100 avian erythrocytes (IF) after a 2-hour action of toxin was equal to 8-9 (IF=8,5%). The same dose of biotoxin (10 mkg/ml) after 4-hours of exposition was inducing intensification of the fusogenic effect. More frequently 3- and 4-nuclear cells were observed. After this stage intensification of fusogenic effect has not been observed. The majority of the double-nuclear cells - dikaryons have the same type of nuclei, so they represented homokaryons. In these cells nuclei had the different size and form (which excludes endomitosis phenomenon). Lower concentrations of *Vipera lebetina* venom (< 5 mkg/ml) the fusogenic effect was not observed. In none of control cases development of homo- or heterokaryons have been observed.

In autoimmune hemolytic anaemias, there are two possibilities of inducing a malignant process: 1) the destructive action of autoimmune antibodies and immunocompetent cells on erythrocytes and their fusogenic effect on these cells and cells of other types, with the possible development of tumor cell; 2) some immunosupressive drugs used in autoimmune states increase considerably the risk of malignant tumors arising, in particular, of non-Hodgkin's lymphoma (B-cell malignancy), in resemblance of cancer of other kind. Besides, the immunosupressive drugs, such as chlorambucil, cyclophosphamide, etc., strongly increase the occurence of chromosomal abnormalities in patients with connective tissue diseases. It is possible that these substances, together with cytolysis of immunocompetent cells, may induce the process of fusion with the formation of a tumorous cell.

Supposing that leucocytes (in this concrete case, lymphocytes and macrophages) are phenotypically dominant cells, their fusion with each other and with other somatic cells may lead to tumor formation of lymphoid and macrophagal nature. Thus, tumorous cells in autoimmune hemolytic anaemias have lymphoid and macrophagal nature. Carcinogenic agents and even infectious viruses and bacterial membranotoxins may induce both fusion and hemolytic effects in somatic cells simultaneously. In autoimmune hemolytic anemias side by side with hemolysis it may take place process of somatic cells fusion with further formation of tumor cells. After bite of snake with hemolytic action of venom together with massive destruction of erythrocytes, there may be induced fusion process of other cellular types with more rigid plasma membranes, with possible development of tumor cell.

Consequently, the fusion of immunocompetent cells with other ones may be regarded as a possible cellular mechanism of malignization in hemolytic anemias of different origin.

CONCLUSION

Exotoxins of definite bacterias are really capable of perforations of target cells plasma membranes. Membranotoxins affect primarily the determinants of plasma membranes, provoke their lysis and, correspondingly, the development of perforations of different size and number in these organoids. A decisive importance in the development of different type, often diametrically opposed pathologies (infections, tumors, etc.) acquires the so-called perforation degree, or the volume or quantity of pores formed in the target-cell plasma membrane by some toxins. In hemolytic anemias of different genesis side by side with hemolysis process of somatic cells fusion process, then karyogamy may take place. After this, it is possible to development of precancerous, and then true cancer cell.

REFERENCES

1. Lancaster, MC. Comparative aspects of aflatoxin-induced hepatic tumors. *Cancer Res.* 1968; 28:2288-2292.
2. Fingerhut, M; Helperin, W; Marlow, D. et al. Cancer mortality in workers exposed to 2,3,7,8-tetrachlorodibenzo-p-dioxin. *N. Engl. J. Med.* 1991; 324:212-218.
3. Parsonnet, J. Bacterial infection as a cause of cancer. *Environ. Health Perspect.* 1995; 103, Suppl. 8:263-268.

4. Lax, AJ. Opinion: bacterial toxins and cancer – a case to answer? *Nat. Rev. Microbiol.* 2005; 3(4):343-349.
5. Vogelman, R; Amieva, MR. The role of bacterial pathogens in cancer. *Curr. Opin. Microbiol.* 2007; 10(1):76-81
6. Travaglione, S; Fabbri, A; Fiorentini, C. The Rho-activating CNF1 toxin from pathogenic E. coli: a risk factor for human cancer development? *Infectious Agents and Cancer.* 2008; 3:4.
7. Caygill, CRJ; Gatenby, PA. *Epidemiology of the association between bacterial infections and cancer.* Springer Science + Business Media B.V. 2012:1-24.
8. Vaananen, P; Kaarianen, L. Fusion and hemolysis of erythrocytes caused by three togaviruses, Semliki Forest, Sindbis and rubella. *J. Gen. Virol.* 1980; 46:467-475.
9. Huang, RT; Rott, R; Klenk, HD. Influenza viruses cause hemolysis and fusion of cells. *Virology.* 1981; 110:243-247.
10. Gogichadze, G; Misabishvili, E; Gogichadze, T. Tumor cell formation by normal somatic cells fusing and cancer prevention prospects. *Med. Hypotheses.* 2006; 66:133-136.
11. Husmann, M; Beckmann, E; Boller, K. et al. Elimination of a bacterial pore-forming toxin by sequental endocytosis and exocytosis. *FEBS Lett.* 2009; 22:337-344.
12. Chang, AH; Parsonnet, J. Role of bacteria in oncogenesis. *Clin. Micr. Reviews.* 2010; 23:837-857.
13. Potez, S; Luginbuhl, M; Monastyrskaya, K. et al. Tailored protection against plasmalemmal injury by annexins with different Ca (2+) sensitivities. *J. Biol. Chemistry.* 2011; 286:17982-17991.
14. Gogichadze, G; Gogichadze, T. *Karyogamic theory of cancer cell formation from the view of the 21st century.* Nova Biomedical Books, New York. 2010.
15. Gogichadze, G. Common characteristics of a cancer cell and logical corroborations of its hybrid essence. *Advances in Genetic Research.* Ed. Kevin V. Urbano. 2011; 46:161-178.
16. Batailler, ER; Klein, B; Durie, BGM. et al. Interrelationship between autoimmunity and B-lymphoid cell oncogenesis in humans. *Clin. Exp. Rheumatol.* 1989; 7:319-328.
17. Lechner, K; Obermeier; HL. Cancer-related microangiopathic hemolytic anemia: clinical and laboratory features in 168 reported cases. *Medicine (Baltimore).* 2012; 91:195-205.

5 LOW PH, AS POSSIBLE REASON OF SPONTANEOUS MALIGNIZATION IN VITRO

In normal and malignized tissues under conditions of active proliferation not infrequently the deterioration of the concentration of hydrogen ions is registered. The pH (potential hydrogen) level measurement in malignant tissues demonstrated that their acid reaction is higher by 0,5 units on the average as compared with normal tissues, although in individual cases pH can deteriorate even by 1-2 units.

In this chapter, we try to establish etiological factors of spontaneously malignized cellular cultures by means of low concentration of hydrogen ions (pH). Currently, it was suggested that the idea about formation of malignant tumors was due exactly to the conditions of low pH [1,2]. On the basis of literary data and our own research, we can conclude that for in cells cultivated *in vitro* (especially in long-term, replacement culturs), one of the most characteristic signs may be considered exact regular reduction of pH, which takes place in the first place during the prolonged and infrequent cellular passages (i.e. seldom replacement of culture, nutrient medium). Up to this time, pH usually reached 6.8 to 6.6 to be followed by desquamation of the greater part of cells from the glass surface and perishing.

Erythrocytes of humans and birds (chickens and pigeons) were used in the experiment as a test-system. The erythrocytes' morhology and their cellular membranes are studied be the light-, phase-contrast- and electron microscopes. During exposition of humans' and birds' erythrocytes in a low pH (6.0 to 5.0) experimental environment (saline), light- and phase-contrast microscopes revealed the lysis of cells and their accumulation in the form of conglomerates. The electron microscopy revealed the homokaryons' formation, also perforation of some erythrocytes' plasma membranes (especially at pH 6.8 to 6.0). This confirmation of ultrastructural analysis is important for fixing the reality of the fusion process. The fusogenic propertis of low pH exponents are clearly revealed in birds' erythrocytes. Besides, as these cells are nuclear, they are on the terminal stage of differentiation and cannot divide. Thus, the processes of fusion, mitosis and endomitosis are not involved.

Based on the above, we concluded that the so-called "spontaneous malignization" of cultivated normal somatic cells is possibly associated with fusion of different (heterokaryons) and homogenous (homokaryons) cellular types, but the possible reason of this process may be cell membranes' local damages (perforations) under conditions of low pH [3].

It is necessary to emphasize that already in 1916, Macklin [4] observed binuclear (dikaryon) and multinucleate (polykaryocytes) cells in a tissue culture. In 1964, Roberts and Cole reported about some mechanisms of formation of polyploid and heteroploid cells in a murine ascites tumor *in vitro* [5]. It turned out that dikaryons may form mononuclear cells by means of fusion of nuclei. Kukain and co-authors (1982) reported about the formation of symplast-like structures in cells' culture of sarcomatous lymph node in cattle [6].

Thus, cultures of normal cells *in vitro* are subjects of spontaneous malignant transformation without the influence of any well-known carcinogenic agents. In our opinion, the etiologic factors of this state may be low pH. On the basis of experiments, we came to the conclusion that low pH turns out to be a sufficiently potent fusogenic agent. A possible reason of the fusion process may be perforations of cell membranes by low pH, which has been experimentally confirmed.

Thus, pH changes can alter the epigenetic and self-correcting mechanisms, accounting for the genetic instability and accumulation of genetic defects seen in malignancy.

CONCLUSION

So-called "spontaneous malignization" of cultivated normal cells is possible associated with fusion of different and homogenous cellular types, but the possible reason of this process may be somatic cells plasma membranes local damages in conditions of low pH. Possible reason of fusion process may be target cells plasma membranes perforations.

REFERENCES

1. Le Boeuf, RF; Kerckaert, GA; Ardema, MJ, et al. Multistage neoplastic transformation of Syrian hamster embryo cells cultured at pH 6.70. *Cancer Res.* 1990; 50:3722-3729.
2. Le Boeuf, RF; Lin, P; Kerckaert, GA. et al. Ultracellular acidification is associated with enhanced morhological transformation in Simian Hamster embryo cells. *Cancer Res.* 1992; 52:144-148.
3. Arvinte, T; Cudd, A; Schulz, B. et al. Low-pH associated of proteins with the membranes of intact red blood cells. II. Studies of the mechanism. *Bioch. Et. Bioph. Acts.* 1989; 98 :61- 68.
4. Macklin, CC. Binucleate and multinucleate cells in tussue cultures. *Anat. Res.* 1916; 10:225.
5. Roberts, DC; Cole, C. Some mechanisms of formation of polyploid and heteroploid cells in a murine ascites tumor in vitro. *J.Natl. Cancer Inst.* 1964; 32:1023-1030.
6. Kukain, DC; Banders, UT; Murovska, MF. Symplasts in cells culture of sarcomatous lymph node of cattle. *Cytologya.* 1982; 8 :9.

6 REASON OF CANCER ARISING ON ALLOTRANSPLANTATIONS

In some cases of allotransplantation, simultaneous development of malignant tumors of different histogenesis (Kaposi's sarcoma, non-Hodgkin's lymphomas, monoblastic sarcomas) may be observed. Whereas usually malignant neoplasms of this histogenesis are just a small share of all tumors, during transplantation of internal organs, they are one of the main types of neoplasms.

Some clinics dealing with problems of transplantology report that recipients with transplanted internal organs (kidneys, skin, bone marrow, etc.) show a significant rise in the incidence of malignant tumor of certain localization and histogenesis [1-3], especially of non-Hodgkin's lymphomas and monoblastic sarcomas. For instance, renal transplanted recipients have 40- to 100-times higher rates on non-Hodgkin's lymphomas and also increased rates of Kaposi's sarcoma. The metastatic prostatic carcionoma was reported in a recipient following heart transplantation.

Transplantation of bone marrow is the most complicated type of this operation, because immune conflict develops in two directions: from host to transplanted bone marrow and from transplanted bone marrow to host ("graft-versus-host reaction"). At the same time, many investigators reported that whole blood and hematopoietic stem cell transplantation was associated with a higher risk of malignant process initiation and relapse. Malignancy has become one of the three major causes of death after allotransplantations. Death from cardio-vascular disease and infection are both decreasing in frequency from a combination of prophylaxis, interventional therapy, etc.

Most recipients of solid organ transplantation receive immunosuppressive therapy for prolonged periods and are at greatly increased risk for tumor development. These tumors have 4 origins: 1.reccurence of malignancies existing in the recipient prior to transplantation; 2.malignancies of recipient origin arising de novo after transplantation. 3.tumors of donor origin arising de novo in the transplanted organ; and 4.pre-existing tumors of donor origin transmitted inadvertently to the recipient via the transplanted organ [4].

Different opinions were given regarding the mechanism of tumor development in these cases: 1. Antigen stimulation. 2.Direct carcinogenetic influence of immunosupressors. 3.Supression of immunity. 4. Activation of endogenous viruses and action of exogenic viruses. Permanent reaction of sensitized donor's lymphocytes against recipient's antigens, i.e., chronic alloantigenic stimulation, is also possible, which may result in lymphoid tissue malignization.

Until recently, the theory of immunological surveillance of F. Burnet (1957) seemed to be the most justified one [5]. However, based on a number of investigation, it may be supposed that immune deficiency is not the necessary condition for the development of malignant tumors and that immune immunocompetence is the consequence rather than the reason for malignant proceses. Old (1981) made the same conclusion on the basis of careful analysis of his own and literature data [6]. At the same time, some aspects of experimental biology and clinical medicine could not be explained in terms of immunological surveillance: for instance, why in chronic "graft-versus-host reaction" (also at transplantation of other internal organs) there developed only lymphoid and macrophagal malignant tumors?

For the first time, we propose to consider malignant tumor formation during allotransplantations of allogenic internal organs in terms of karyogamic theory of carcinogenesis [7]. Experience in transplantology tentatively testifies that even in cases of maximal antigen compatibility of donors and recipients, immune conflict is unavoidable. As we believe, in immunological conflict between recipient and donor cells, which is inevitable even under careful selection, the process of cells' destruction in some cases may be accompanied by damages of plasma membranes and somatic hybridization between immunocompetent cells of the recipient and any cell of transplanted donor's tissue (graft). This occurence may lead to the emergence of a tumorous cell, synkaryon. Unlike autohybridization, where tumorous cells may be formed during fusion of somatic cells of the same organism, in allotransplantations, one may speak about allo (homo) hybridization.

As it is shown, the macro organism reacts to the allotransplantant by development of humoral and cellular immune responses (immune cytolysis). In the development of transplantation immunity the most important roles are played by specific antibodies and T-killer (cytotoxic) cells (immune effectors). 1. Antibody molecules have 2 main functions: they bind to the immunogenic antigens (in this case they are represnted by superficial antigens of the allotransplantant cells) and after interaction with the antigen initiates involvement of different cells and molecules. The constant region (C region) of the antibodies defines the type of the response after the antibody-antigen interaction, whether this is complement-mediated lysis, cellular cytotoxicity, enhanced phagocytosis, etc. 2.Transplantational cellular immune responce is conducted by T-cytotoxic cells: after the sensitization of the recipient by the donor antigens the killer cells are migrating to the transplant tissue and are having inducing the cytotoxic effect. It is known that cytotoxic T-killer cells are causing the damage to the target cells by production of the different molecules (perforines, granzymes, etc.). In the presence of calcium, perforines interact with the plasmatic membrane of the target cells and after the polymerization they are forming the transmembrane channels (pores) in this organoid. So both antibodies and cytotoxic cells can induce damages (perforations) of different degree on somatic cells plasma membranes, which can represent the precancerous and later the true cancerous cells formation.

Besides, since lymphoid tissue cells as a well as macrophages are the morphological substrate ensuring the formation of the immune response to antigenic stimulation, cells of this type may be one of the essential objects in fusion during organ allotransplantation, especially as the process of contact and penetration of lymphocytes to other cells in immunological conflict ("peripolesis" and "emperipolesis", respectively), as well as facts of fusion of macrophages with other cells are well known [8]. In a case when macrophages and lymphocytes cultivated together, lymphocytes move around macrophages and formed so-called rosettes (peripolesis). During this process, lymphocytes inculcate their appendixes into cytoplasm of macrophages and in some cases make root in these cells (emperipolesis). Specifically, what does the mechanism of malignant conversion consist in, in the case of allotrasplantations?

In our opinion, tumorous cells represent a hybrid, the so-called tumorous synkaryon, emerging as a result of the fusion of two normal somatic cells. Stem cells, fibroblasts, macrophages, lymphoid cells, undifferentiated cells of various tissues and others show an increased capability to create viable hybrids. In case of allotransplantation, during the perforation of cellular membranes induced by antibodies or T-killers, the total charge of plasma membranes changes, and the cells acquire the capability of closely approaching (adhesion), which frequently, especially upon coincidence of the perforated parts, may serve as a prerequisite to fusion process. In result of this, may form dikaryons _ heterokaryons (cells with nuclei of different type of cells) or homokaryons (cells with homogenous nuclei) in the process of fusion with one another or with other cells, and then, in case of synchronous mitosis or mechanical reunification of nuclei, they may form synkaryons (mononuclear hybrid cells), with tetraploid or hypoteteraploid sets of chromosomes on initial stage of hybridization. The forming hybrid synkaryon (so-called synkaryon of stage I) is an initiated, i.e., precancerous cell may exist in the corresponding tussue for a long time, sometimes even several decades. On the promotion stage, after the influence of complete (full) carcinogens or promoters on tissue, where precancerous synkaryons pre-exist, in precancerous cells, the chromosomal aberrations of different types and genes amplifications may arise. From the chromosomal aberrations, the most dangerous in carcinogenic respect are nonbalanced translocations, and also duplications. This event usully leads to genes' amplification. Following the above-marked conversion on the sub-cellular and molecular levels, there may arise true tumorous synkaryon (synkaryon of stage II), malignant cell with the ability of uncontrolled proliferation.

In the fusion process, the highest activity may be shown by recipient's macrophages and T-lymphocytes, which are effector cells against tissue incompatibility antigens. On the basis of the above and taking into consideration the fact that lymphocytes and macrophages are dominant cells also with respect to phenotypic properties, in the most cases of tumors, malignant cells, which develop during allogenic organ transplantations, may have lymphoid (T- or B-cell), macrophagal or the so-called "intermediate" morphology.

I.e. in the case of allotransplantations, cancer cells' formation more frequently could be originated from donor (graft) cells rather than from the recipient's own cells. Although in some cases fusogeny may occur between immunocompetent cells of the recipient or between last cells and any of transplanted donor's (graft) cells.

Transplantation of allogenic internal organs in some cases may also promote relapse of tumor process, especially in myelotransplantation to patient with leukemia at the clinical and hematological remission stage, or to persons with still unrevealed, "dormant" malignant tumor or leukemia. Since transplanted hemopoietic cells of the bone marrow, in accordance will the well-known "homing" mechanism, settle in their habitual sites, i.e., in various parts of recipient's bone marrow formation of a malignant cell, possibly with new geno- and phenotypical properties may be expected.

In our opinion, the mechanism of relapse or progression of tumor process may be also due to somatic hybridization of recipient's tumorous cells with transplanted normal bone marrow or other internal organ's cells, especially as one cannot exclude an increased somatic hybridization ability of tumorous cells. On the other hand, data on prediction of results of tumorous cells' fusion with normal or other tumorous cells are very contradictory. As shown by numerous investigations, malignancy is some cases is a dominant and in other cases a recessive trait [9,10].

Confirmation of proposition about fusion of tumorous cells with normal cells in transplantation of allogenic internal organs may be experimental observations of some scientists. In particular, these scientists injected cells of human tumors into hamsters and revealed that tumorous cells fused spontaneously with recipients' normal cells and formed tumorous hybrid cells with a new geno- and phenotypic properties. For example, Fialkow and co-authors (1971) and also Thomas and co-authors (1972) reported about leukemia relapse in two girls after total radiation and following transplantation of healthy brothers' bone marrow. Relapse of leukemia was marked after prolonged remission _ from 62 and 153 days, accordingly [11,12]. Leukemia cells were donor-derived, i.e. had lymphoblastoid cells' morphology and karyogrammes of man type. Both donors continued to be healthy. It was also shown [13], that in transplantation of bone marrow to leukemia patient, donor cells occasionally may hybridize with leukemia cells of recipient, as a result of which, new tumorous synkaryons are formed. Besides, Witherspoon and co-authors (1985) reported about the case when leukemia relapse took place more than six years after bone marrow transplantation [14]. The donor and the recipient in this case were of the same sex and had no cytogenetic differences. Nevertheless, DNA analysis revealed that leukemia cells were of the donor type.

On the other hand, increased risk of malignant tumors in allotransplanted recipients may be induced by cyclosporine A, too, which usually is applied for immune forces inhibition: in allotransplantations, in autoimmune reactions and against tumor process. Moreover, carcinogenic [15,16] and teratogenic effects of this substance [17] was established. Along with this it should be also mentioned that before 70-80 ths of the XX century or before the use of cyclosporine A in allotransplantant patients, occurrence of the cancerous formations in the recipients was almost of the same frequency as for the cases of other immunodepressants (e.g. azatioprine, prednisolone, ionizing and other types of radiation and also the antilymphocytic medicines) were used.

Thus, in transplantations of different allogenic internal organs, bone marrow, and even transfusion of blood and its components (e.g. leukocytes), and hematopoietic stem cells, physicians should take into consideration the likely probability of serious complications due to the emergence of tumorous cells in non-oncological recipients and relapse or progression of malignant process in tumor-carriers.

6.1 Cancer cell formation by immune cytolysis

It has been established that some people's serum (antibodies) provokes agglutination (contact, adhesion) of cells, which should seemingly be caused by disintegration (perforation) of the respective cell plasmalemma, as a result of reduction of an electric charge on the surface of these cells, further contact and adhesion. The contact, adhesion of somatic cells may be closely related to the development of a cancer cell.

In addition to a specific effect of different pathogens (viruses, bacterial toxins, biotoxins of other types and so on) on the plasma membrane of the target cells, being reflected in the formation of perforations of different number and size quantity, approximately the same effect can be characteristic of the so-called immune (both cell-immune and humor-immune) cytolysis.

Immunocytolysis is one of the major mechanisms ensuring a rapid destruction of virus-infected cells and the virus neutralization. As known, 2 radically different forms of immune cytolysis are distinguished: cell-immune and humor-immune cytolysis.

1) In the first case, the object of attacks by immune (effector) killer cells, including T-lymphocytes, become the virus antigen-containing target-cells, which can result in immunocytolysis. Thus, the cell-immune cytolysis is carried out directly by the killer (cytotoxic) cells. The killing can be performed except T-lymphocytes, by activated macrophages, natural killers (NK), and other cells. Killers perform their functions either from a distance or when in contact with the target cell. The killers generate substances of cytotoxic and cytolytic action, causing thus cell necrosis with disintegration of its plasmalemma or induction of apoptosis. The cytotoxic effect of killers is realized in the target cell plasmalemma by special proteins – perforins which lead to the formation in this organoid of perforations (pores). Perforins (together with granzymes and granulolyzins) are localized in killer cells (macrophages, T-lymphocytes, NK-cells) granules. The killer-excreted perforin molecules after being inserted in the target cell plasmalemma are polymerized, forming pores in this organoid which can, in the case of great number or size, induce the cell destruction or other cytopathogenic effects.

2) In the case of humor-immune cytolysis, the target cell plasmalemma together with the complement is directly attacked by antibodies. This type of cytolysis occurs in the cells infected with rubella, herpes simplex, ortho- and paramyxoviruses, lymphocytic choriomeningitis, tick-born encephalities and so on. The essence of said occurrence consists in the cell strucure injury by specific ntibodies of viral and cellular antigens. This may lead to mthe

formation in the plasma membranes of target cells of pores, a two- threefold increase in the cell size, the nucleus transfer to the periphery, and finally the complement-mediated lysis of the cell. The degeneration or dissolution of cells caused by the disruption of plasma membrane takes place.

The target cell killing is carried out in several stages: 1) killer-target-cell contact; 2) killer activation; 3) exocytosis of toxic substances by the killer; and 4) toxic effect on the target cell. Thus, pore-forming enzyme, antibodies, peptids, etc. cause plasma membrane damage in target cells, with consequences as diverse as proliferation or cell destruction [18].

CONCLUSION

In immunological conflict between recipient and donor cells, the process of cell's destruction in some cases may be accompanied by damages of plasmalemma and somatic hybridization between immunocompetent cells of the recipient and any cell of transplanted donor's tissue, which may lead to the emergence of a tumor cells. Same mechanism is observed in case of immune cytolysis.

REFERENCES

1. Penn, I. De novo malignancy in pediatric organ transplant recipients. *J.Pediatr. Surg.* 1994; 29:221-226.
2. Swinnen, LJ. Diagnosis and treatment of transplant-related lymphoma. *Ann. Oncol.* 2000; 11:45-48.
3. Fiedor, P; Wierbicki, Z; Pawelec, K. et al. Human papillomavirus as a risk factor for development of cancer in allograft recipients. *Ann. Transplantology. Index Copernicus J. abstract.* 2009; 14 (Suppl.1):24.
4. Gazdar, Adi F. Tumors arising after organ transplantation sorting out their origins. *JAMA.* 1997; 277 (2):154-155.
5. Burnet, F.M. Cancer _ a biological approach. *Brit. Med. J.* 1957; 17 :779-793.
6. Old, L.J. Cancer immunology: the search for specifity _ G.H.A. Clowes memorial lecture. *Cancer Res.*1981; 41:361-375.
7. Gogichadze, G; Gogichadze, T. *Karyogamic theory of cancer cell formation from the view of the XXI century.* Nova Biomedical Books, New York. 2010.
8. Munzarova, M; Kovaric, J. Is cancer a macrophage-mediated autoagressive disease? *Lancet.* 1987; 1:952-954.
9. Harris, H. The analysis of malignancy by cell fusion: the position in 1988. *Cancer Res.* 1988; 48:3302-3306.
10. De Baetselier, P. *Neoplastic progression by somatic cell fusion.* Influence Tumor Drv. Host._ Dodrecht, etc. 1989.
11. Fialkow, PJ; Thomas, ED; Bryant, JD. et al. Leukemic transformation of engrafted human marrow cells in vivo. *Lancet.* 1971; 1 :251.

12. Thomas, ED; Bryant, JI; Buckner, CD, et al. Leukemic transformation of engrafted human marrow cells in vivo. *Lancet.* 1972; 1:1310.
13. Von Heiden, HW; Moore, GE. Hypothesis: engrafted human bone marrow and blood cells in culture. *Blood.* 1972; 40:754-758.
14. Witherspoon, RP; Schubach, W; Neiman, P. et al. Donor cell leukemia developing six years after marrow grafting for acute leukemia. *Blood.* 1985; 65:1172-1174.
15. Frei, U; Bode, U; Repp, H. et al. Malignancies under cyclosporine after kidney transplantation: analysis of a 10-year period. *Transplant. Proc.* 1993; 25 (1Pt 2):1394-1396.
16. Vakeva, L; Reitamo, S; Pukkala, E. et al. Long-term follow-up of cancer risk in patients treated with short-term cyclosporine. *Acta Derm. Venereol.* .2008; 88:117-120.
17. Penn, I. Cancers following cyclosporine therapy. *Transplantation.* 1987; 43:32-35.
18. Babiychuk, EB; Monastyrskaya, K; Potez, S. et al. Intracellular Ca2+ operates a switch between repair and lysis of streptolysin 0-perforated cells. *Cell Death and Differentiation.* 2009; 16:1126-1134.

7 SOME "BIOLOGICAL NONSENSES" FROM THE POSITION OF THE KARYOGAMIC THEORY OF CARCINOGENESIS

One rather important remark should be made around this chapter. The main theses of this chapter, with insignificant modifications, are stated in the monographs published in New York in 2010 and then in Saarbrucken in 2013. We repeat it because this chapter seems rather important to us: there expressed an assumption about the cellular and sub-cellular mechanisms of tumor formation by the effect of some fatty acid, carbohydrate and, most important, of distilled water. The experimental tumors caused by distilled water and physiological solution have long been known as the so-called "biological nonsenses" and the explanation of these facts by the other, currently most popular theories of carcinogenesis, has been found impossible. Thus, the repetition of this chapter (with minor amendments) is conditioned by focusing attention of the interested reader on this problem.

Malignant transformation of the normal somatic cells into cancer ones can be assisted by the very difference in their nature agents and factors: penetrating radiation of different nature, numerous chemical carcinogens, some oncogenic and infectious viruses, some pharmacological agents, some kinds of irritation, etc. The above-enumerated carcinogens are probably initiating some common mechanism of conversion of normal cells into transformed state.

In experimental oncology, examples are known on induction of malignant neoplasms in laboratory animals after inoculation with indifferent at first sight substances, such as some fatty acids, carbohydrates, physiological solution (NaCl), even distilled water, etc. The similar results were obtained after an epidemiological research of some of these agents, e.g. in respect of dietary fats and carbohydrates.

In this chapter we make an attempt to explain the essence of these occurrences by means of karyogamic theory of carcinogenesis.

7.1 Induction of malignant tumors by some fatty acids

The relationship of nutrition and cancer is not a new concern. For instance, as long ago as 1809 Lambe published dietary recommendations for cancer prevention. Hoffman (1915) suggested that excessive weight and high caloric intake might be at the root of the increased cancer incidence in the developed world [1]. Recent data refer to the influence of a restricted diet on the incidence of radiation induced tumors and leukemia in rats and mice [2]. The incidence of malignant tumors developing in rats and mice of either sex, exposed to total-body gamma irradiation, was reduced considerably.

During the period of rapid development of civilization, on a relatively short evolutionary scale of time, nourishment of humans underwent deep changes. Physiology of a human being of the Stone Age is in confrontation with the nourishment of the 20th-21st centuries. After industrialization of the society and growth of its economics state, the ratio of dietary fats in human diets relatively increased in the form of meat and vegetable oils.

Some aspects of fatty acids interrelation with the process of carcinogenesis scientists interested long time ago. Correlation between dietary fats consumption and development of breast cancer was first observed in early 20s of the 20th century. In the late 30s, new data on the carcinogenetic properties of several fatty acids after their overheating appeared in the scientific literature [3,4]. There are number of experimental data on the origin of malignant tumors of stomach and liver in mice and rats being fed by overheated dietary fats for a long time. These authors demonstrated the development of stomach and liver papillomas, cancers and sarcomas in mice after feeding them cotton oil, which was heated during 4 hours at $350^{o}C$. The similar results were obtained after feeding mice with cholesterol, turpentine, orange, eucalyptus and croton oils (this last substance is the well-known promoter, which possess very weak carcinogenic properties too).

Intensive experiments of this kind were conducted in the current years. In experiments in mice and rats etiologic role of dietary fats in producing malignant tumors of different histogenesis and localization, in particular, breast, colon and prostate cancers were confirmed [5,6]. In experiments in laboratory animals it was demonstrated that high content of dietary fats in food (40% of calories), stimulated development of breast cancer, but rations with low content of dietary fats (10% of calories) did not reveal carcinogenic effect. At the same time it was demonstrated that polyunsaturated fatty acids increase process of carcinogenesis more intensively, than saturated fatty acids. Tumors arise when ration consists of polyunsaturated fatty acids and do not occur if monounsaturated fatty acids are present therein [6].

The importance of several dietary fats in producing malignant tumors is also testified by the data of epidemiological analysis, by the method of case-control [7,8].

At the same time, some scientists report on the fusogenic effect of different (but not all!) fatty acids in tissue culture *in vitro* [9-11]. In these works numerous fatty acids were studied for their fusogenic properties. These scientists concluded that the fusion process proceeds most easily in the case of unsaturated fatty acids. Various degrees of cells' fusion were seen with linoleic, undecylenic, myristoleic, palmitoleic acids and glyceryl monooleate. In this connection, of interest is to mention the already confirmed fact that although the glyceryl monooleate induces intensive fusogeny, the glyceryl dioleate induces only agglutination (not fusion), whereas glyceryl trioleate induces neither fusion nor agglutination prcesses.

Fusion process apparently does not occur with several saturated fatty acids, for example, with caproic, caprylic fatty acids etc. Though some saturated fatty acids still induce process of cells' fusion (especially C10, C11, C12, C13, C14 saturated fatty acids).

The mechanism inducing malignant neoplasms by these substances in human is so far unknown. Explanation of this mechanism on the basis of such famous modern theories of carcinogenesis, as polyetiologic, virus- genetic, oncogenes and so on, is impossible. But parallelism between carcinogenicity and fusogeny of these substances, allow us to consider this phenomenon as confirmation of somatic hybridization theories of carcinogenesis.

On the basis of literature data and our own experimental observations we make attempt to explain the carcinogenicity of some dietary fats from the standpoint of hybridization theory of carcinogenesis (in particular, from theory of "two synkaryons"). In experimental conditions we verified fusogenic abilities of some saturated and unsaturated fatty acids and carried out comparative research their influence on cellular membranes.

Our experiments established that polyunsaturated (linoleic) and monounsaturated (oleic) fatty acids differ from saturated acids by a high intensity of interaction with cellular membranes. Much importance during fusogeny was also given to the fusogeny index (FI). Especially high fusogenic activity was revealed by the oleic acid. However, the epidemiological analysis failed to detect the carcinogenic activity of this fatty acid. What is the reason of this strange occurrence? A reverse correlation between fusogenic and carcinogenic abilities has been revealed: the higher is the fusogenic activity of this or that substance, the lower is its carcinogenic activity and vice versa. In particular, in the case of high fusogenic ability of a substance (e.g., the oleic acid) the formation of unviable giant polykaryocytes is induced and carcinogenic effect is less manifested; and vice versa, the carcinogenic effect is higher in the presence of low fusogenic ability of the substance (e.g., the linoleic acid) because of the formation of mainly dikaryons with high oncogenic potency [12,13].

Thus, a tumor cell is a result of fusion of two normal somatic cells under the effect of certain carcinogenic (fusogenic) agents. Dikaryons (hetero- or homokaryons) are formed at the stage of initiation, and then following the reunion of nuclei – mononuclear, tetraploid (or sub-tetraploid) initiated cells, i.e. precancerous synkaryon (synkaryon of stage I). At the stage of promotion, after the carcinogens or promoters have influenced the corresponding tissues (with pre-existence of precancerous cells) the intensity of cell's proliferation is induced. This cell (precancerous cell), after some conversions on a molecular and sub-cellular levels, may be transformed into a tumor synkaryon (synkaryon of stage II).

Ahkong et al. (1973) explain the fusogeny process by an increase in the permeability of plasma membranes of the target cells, but refrain from elucidating the concrete mechanism of this phenomenon [12]. In our opinion, the permeability increase of the plasma membranes is associated with the plasmalemma structure changes. In other words, the permeability growth should be in direct relation with the development of perforations in this organoid. A perforation may, in turn, precondition fusogeny only on condition that pores are not of very large size (which will necessarily lead to the destruction of cells) and, most important, the coincidence of the perforated sections of the neighbor cells' plasmalemma takes place. In case the pores of large volume (size) are produced, the abnormally high permeability might occur in the plasma membranes, because of which they can no longer be reparated and the cell deteriorates.

Certain dietary fats may induce perforations of definite size or modifications of plasma membranes of somatic cells under several conditions. This may be premise for cells' fusion and hetero- and homokaryons formation. At the same time it is possible that the movement of proteins, glycoproteins and lipids take place on the membranes of somatic cells. This evidence may also play a definite role in the process of fusion.

A prolonged action of some dietary fats (if they possess promoter abilities too) or other carcinogens and promoters on the corresponding tissue induce the formation of the first tumor cell, synkaryon of stage II.

The experimental data show that, as a rule, the penetration of certain substances into cells (in case their molecule size exceeds that of glycerin molecule size) takes place after getting through the lipid bilayer of plasmalemma. This assumption testifies also the fact that the penetration of substances into a cell is in correlation with its lipophilic (hydrophobic) abilities.

The fatty acids' molecules have a double nature – hydrophilic and hydrophobic (the correlation with them depends on pH). This ability of fatty acids is similar to that of detergents. The penetration of fatty acids into a cell may begin following the interaction of their hydrophobic parts with the lipid parts of the plasmalemma. This interaction may induce some damages in plasmalemma ultrastructure and its transition into the metastable state. These favorable conditions may be a reason of the fusion of cellular membranes.

Thus, based on the data of our and other scientists' experiments and theoretical judgments, it is possible to conclude that some fatty acids possess the initiating abilities, i.e. the ability to form initiated, precancerous cells (synkaryons of stage I). Given that some other scientists have also identified the promotional effects of fatty acids [6], certain fatty acids are likely to possess the properties of perfect (full) carcinogens.

7.2 Possible reason of induction of malignant tumors by some carbohydrates

Population of so-called "developing" countries 80% of calories receive from cereals, which consist of complex carbohydrates. After the industrialization of countries and development of their economics, in the ration of population's part of fats (meat and vegetable oil) rise considerably. At the same time consumption of refined sugar (simple carbohydrate) increases too. After such changes in nutrition among the population occurrence of breast, colon and colorectal cancers rise.

In 1935 and 1938 Nishiyama, who studied the carcinogenic properties of several chemical substances in rats, subcutaneously inoculated carbohydrates, in particular, glucose, together with certain substances (orthoaminoazotoluol). These experiments [14,15] demonstrated that upon daily inoculation of 25% glucose solution (1g/kg) for more than 200 days, polymorphocellular sarcomas were developed in the sites of injection, in five cases out of seven. Malignant tumors used to occur in most cases after increasing the glucose concentrations.

These experiments were improved by the studies of Takizawa (1940). Takizawa subcutaneously inoculated into mice 25% glucose solution daily [16]. In 250 days of such inoculations spindle-cell sarcomas started to form in the sites of injection in 5 mice out of 18. The tumors so formed were passed to the healthy mice. Tumors used to develop in rats and mice also upon prolonged subcutaneous inoculation of other carbohydrate solution. In these experiments, in the sites of injection of 25% fructose solution sarcomas were formed in 2 mice out of 16, and in 4 mice out of 13 in the site of inoculation by 25% galactose solution.

In 1956 the similar results were received by Azakawa [17].

In 1957, Takizawa, Ooguchi and Hayashi observed the development of sarcoma in 1 out of 20 mice, following the daily subcutaneous injection of 0.5 ml of 25% maltose solution [18].

Mettlin and Piver (1990), Harlow and co-authors (1991) by an epidemiological analysis with the case-control study established that milk consumption increased the risk of ovary cancer because of an association of lactose with ovary failure [19,20]. Moreover, by an epidemiologic analysis the direct association between the colorectal and breast cancers and intake of refined carbohydrates [21-23] was found . The mechanism of the colorectal cancer development in this concrete case the authors explained by the so-call insulin/colon cancer hypothesis.

Several articles reported that after the inoculation of chemical carcinogens in rats, rations of which were enriched by starch, breast tumors developed in considerably less cases than in animals, the ration of which was enriched by dextrose (the simple sugar) instead of starch.

The mechanism of influence of these classes of carbohydrates (dextrose, glucose, fructose et al) on the experimental carcinogenesis is yet unknown.

In scientific literature there are only few data on the possible fusogenic action of several sugars. In 1917 Kalashnikov studied the action of glucose solution on spawn of perch [24]. He observed giant syncytiums consisting of parablasts and fusing with them of free blastomeres. There are many nuclei in syncytium in resting phase or dividing by means of amitosis. Author assumed that in some cases fusion of several nuclei into one does occur.

It was shown that hybridization of somatic cells promoted by sucrose [10].

Recently Smeland and Funderud [25] have reported about the possible interrelation of the cellular adhesion induced by sugar molecules and the tumor arising.

In the last years, some authors have reported about the fusogenic activity of glucose, lactose, fructose, with the exception of starch [13].

The above-mentioned correlation between the fusogenic and carcinogenic properties of several carbohydrates may indicate that following the effect of glucose, galactose and maltose in Nishyama's and Takizawa's experiments malignant tumors may arise by means of somatic cells fusion and further hybridization.

The effect of some carbohydrates on the cell's glycocalix and plasma membranes may induce perforations or modifications of these components under corresponding conditions. This may be a reason of the cell's further fusion and the formation of dikaryons (homo- and heterokaryons), and then precancerous cells, and true tumor synkaryons.

7.3 Induction of malignant tumors by distilled water

As was shown after experimental works of Warabioka (1956; 1957), Watanabe and his co-authors (1957) the daily inoculation of distilled water into intraperitoneal cavity of rats, in some cases development of connective tissue malignant tumors – sarcomas, in particular, fibrosarcomas, maybe induced [26-28]. For instance, in experiments of Watanabe, in 2 rats after daily inoculation of 3 ml of distilled water, during 15-17 months fibrosarcomas were observed, which in one case was transplantable. Warabioka, in 13 months after daily injection of distilled water, in 1 rat observed sarcoma, which at lethal stage reached the size of a hen's egg.

Inoculation of 1%, 1,5% or 2% aqueous solution of trypan blue injected subcutaneously in the Wistar or Sprague-Dawley rats (0,5 ml per 150 g body weight, fortnightly) induced production of hepatic sarcomas [26].

Interpretation of these results from the position of different theories and hypotheses of carcinogenesis, turn out to be impossible. For example, it is difficult to express, how distilled water can activate some endogenous cancer viruses or induce expression of definite oncogenes with the following development of malignant neoplasms.

At the first sight it is complicated to explain these events from the position of theory of "two synkaryons" too, such as the fusogenic properties of distilled water are unknown yet.

On the other hand it is known, that in some conditions distilled water has the capability to induce destruction of somatic cells, in particular, erythrocytes plasma membranes, what is followed by the intensive hemolysis. Distilled water in cells with more rigid plasma membranes (leucocytes, fibroblasts and so on) may induce smaller, reparable perforations in neighbouring cells, which frequently, especially upon coincidence of the perforated parts of plasma membranes, may serve as a prerequisite to fusion process.

To isolate leukocyte layer (buffy coat) from the whole blood for electron microscopic research and for other purpose, a method of the so-called "hypotonic shock" was used [29].

The essence of this method consists in addition of distilled water to the whole blood with anticoagulant substances (for example, heparin), with ratio of 1:1, following shaking up during 15 seconds. In this period of time intensive hemolysis with the destruction of absolute majority of erythrocytes with retaining of intact leucocytes is observed. At the same time in last case does not exclude more or less considerable damages (but not ruptures) of the leucocytes plasma membranes or form of pores of little size.

As has been noted above, any fusogenic factors may induce perforations of definite size or modifications of cells' plasma membranes with the follow-up fusion of cellular membranes. Perforations of big size induce a considerable destruction of cytoplasmic membranes, cytolysis and perishing of the cells.

Based on the above, we may assume that daily injections of distilled water into the intraperitoneal cavity (or subcutaneously) of experimental animals may in some cases induce the perforations of different size of neighboring cells' plasma membranes, which sometimes assist their approaching and follow-up fusion.

Confirmation of above-mentioned may be data of Sokolov (1955), in which at research of seminal glands of some insects, in particular, of *Omocestus viridilus* L., *Chorthippus albomarginatus* D.C. and *Ch. parallelus* Zett., injection of distilled water took place [30]. This manipulation revealed giant polynuclear cellular structures formed after the fusion of normal cells and their nuclei. These giant cells, are as a rule, subject to deterioration.

One may think that in the sites of inoculation (or near them) distilled water may induce in cellular plasma membranes perforations of big size, which from the oncological point of view are not dangerous. And only in the tissues localized little far from the site of inoculation the conditions (perforations of plasmalemmas) favorable for cells' approaching, their fusion and follow-up somatic hybridization with arising of precancerous synkaryon are formed.

The perishing of a considerable quantity of somatic cells as a result of plasma membranes' destruction directly on the site of injection is known to be favorable for the process of regeneration of the corresponding tissue and intensive proliferation of cells (by production of the "growth factor"). This may in turn also involve the process of precancerous synkaryons' proliferation. Precancerous cells, subject to some processes on the molecular and sub-cellular levels, may be transformed into a tumor synkaryon (synkaryon of stage II).

7.4 Induction of malignant neoplasms by physiological solution (NaCL)

Some data of scientific literature testify the carcinogenic action of a physiological solution (saline) under experimental conditions. In 1940 a Japanese scientist Tokoro reported on the development of reticulosarcoma and spindle-cell sarcoma in the site of daily subcutaneous injection of 5-20% physiological solution (saline) in two rats [31]. A malignant tumor in the first rat developed after 97 injections, and in second rat – after 82 injections.

The said report is so far the only one (with the exception of data by J. Weisburger, E. Weisburger [32]) and this fact cannot be explained by the existing theories and hypotheses of carcinogenesis.

The explaining of this phenomenon by the karyogamic theory of carcinogenesis is also difficult because in literature there is extremely little data on fusogenic properties of this substance. However, in 1917 Kalashnikov observed a giant syncytium with many nuclei in the rest phase and during division when he acted on spawn of perch by physiological solution [24]. The main cause in this process, to the author's opinion, is amitosis and fusion of several nuclei.

As has been shown by the some researchers in the last years, saline may under some conditions modify the properties of cytoplasmic membranes' lipid bilayer. This may ultimately induce alterations of the negative charge of somamtic cells' surface, which may assist to the approaching of cells and as a result – their fusion.

The parallelism between the carcinogenic and fusogenic properties of a physiological solution (although on the basis of individual observations) allows us to assume the mechanism of its action. Thus, this strange fact we may explain by means of karyogamic ("two synkaryons") theory of carcinogenesis.

CONCLUSION

In the experimental oncology there are number of examples on the induction of malignant neoplasms in the laboratory animals after the inoculation, at first sight, of indifferent, non-carcinogenic substances, such as dietary fats, carbohydrates, distilled water, physiological solution, etc. It is possible that some dietary fats and carbohydrates too may induce perforations or modifications of somatic cell's plasma membranes under some conditions. This fact plays a definite role in the process of fusion and in forming tumor cells. Distilled water and saline have the ability of destroying somatic cell's plasma membranes. Perforations of this organoid are the reason of cellular membranes' fusion. The daily injections of distilled water and saline into laboratory animals may induce perforations of plasma membranes, which assist their approaching and subsequent fusion.

REFERENCES

1. Hoffman, FL. *The mortality from cancer throughout the world. Newark*: Prudential, 1915.
2. Gross, L. Inhibition of the development of tumors or leukemia in mice and rats after reduction of food intake. *Cancer. Res.* 1988; 62:1463-1465.
3. Beck, S. Sarcoma produces by subcutaneous injections of overheated cotton-seed oil into mice. *Brit J. Exper Pathol.* 1941; 22:299-302.
4. Roffo, AH. Accion cancerigena de los derivados fenantrenicos del colesterol. *Bol Inst De Med Exper Para el Estud y Trat d Cancer.* 1938; 15:837-845.
5. Freedman, LS; Clifford, C; Messina, M. Analysis of dietary fat, calories, body weight, and the development of mammary tumors in rats and mice: a review. *Cancer Res.* 1990; 50: 5710-5719.
6. Rao, CV; Hirose, Y; Indranie, C. et al. Modulation of experimental colon tumorigenesis by types and amounts of dietary fatty acids. *Cancer Res.* 2001; 61:1927- 1933.
7. Lucy, JA; Ahkong QF; Cramp, FC. et al. Cell fusion without viruses. *Biochem J.* 1971; 124: 46-47.
8. Cohen, LA; Thompson, DO; Maeura, Y. Dietary fat and mammary cancer. I. Promoting effect of different dietary fats on N-nitrosomethylurea-induced rat mammary tumorigenesis. *J Natl Cancer Inst.* 1986; 77:33-42.
9. Smith-Warner, SA; Spiegelman, D; Adami, HO. Types of dietary fat and breast cancer: a pooled analysis of cohort studies. *Intern. J. Cancer.* 2001; 92: 767-774.
10. Ahkong, QF; Cramp, FC; Fischer, D. et al. Studies on chemically induced cell fusion. *J. Cell Sci.* 1972; 10: 769-787.
11. Ahkong, QF; Fischer, D; Tampion, W. et al. Mechanisms of cell fusion. *Nature.*1975; 253:194-195.
12. Gogichadze, G; Beniashvili, D; Piriashvili, V. et al. Some aspects of interaction of dietary fats and carcinogenesis. *Proc. Acad. Sciences of Georgia (seria biol).* 1994; 20:69-74.
13. Gogichadze, GK., Gogichadze, TG. Cancer as a result of somatic cells fusion caused by some dietary fats and carbohydrates. *Med. Hypotheses.* 2005; 65:622- 623.
14. Nishiyama, Y. Experimentalle hepatombildung durch futterung mit 0- aminoazotoluol bei maus. *Gann.*1935; 29:285-294.
15. Nishiyama, Y. Experimentalle erzeugung des sarkoms bei ratten durch wiered- holte injectionen von glucoselosung. *Gann.* 1938; 32: 85-98.
16. Takizawa, N. Experimentalle erzeugung des sarkoms bei der maus durch die injektion-von glucose, fructose und galactose. Ein beitrag zur frage der histogenese des fibroplastischelen sarkoma.*Gann.*1940; 34:1-5.
17. Takizawa, N; Ooguchi, H; Hayashi, J. Experimental production of sarcoma in mice with administration of reducing saccharides, especially maltose and some effects of adenosine triphosphate on the sarcomatous proliferation of fibroblasts induced by injection of reducing saccharides. *Gann.* 1957; 48:556-558.

18. Azakawa, S. Experimental production of sarcoma of mice with the subcutaneous high concentrated sugar solution, especially lactose, and mixture of laevulose and glucose. *Gann.* 1956; 47:592-593.
19. Mettlin, CJ., Piver MS. A case-control study of milk drinking and ovarian cancer risk. *Amer. J. Epidemiol..* 1990; 132:871-876.
20. Harlow, BL; Craemer, DW; Geller, J. The influence of lactose consumption on the association of oral contraceptive use and ovarian cancer risk. *Amer. J. Epidemiol.* 1991; 134: 445-453.
21. Franceschi, S; Del Maso, L; Augustin, L. Dietary glycemic load and colorectal cancer risk. *Ann. Oncol.* 2001; 12: 172-178
22. Hassan, AB; Macaulay, VM. The insulin-like growth factor system as a therapeutic target in colorectal cancer. *Ann. Oncol.* 2002; 13:349-356.
23. Key, TG. Glycemic index, hyperinsulinemia, and breast cancer risk. *Ann. Oncol.* 2001; 12:1507-1509.
24. Kalashnikov, PP. Observations over development of eggs of Persa fluviatillis in artificial solutions. *Works of Soc. Natural Scientists of Petrograd.* 1917; XLV-LII.
25. Smeland, EB; Funderud, S. Sugar molecules, cell adhesion and cancer etiology. *Tidsskrift. Nor Laegeforen.* 1992; 112:2834.
26. Warabioka, K. On the experimentally induced subcutaneous sarcoma in the rat following repeated topical injections of aqua distillata gelida. *Gann.* 1956; 47: 603-606.
27. Warabioka, K. On the induction of sarcoma in rats injected with aqua distillata gelida. Second report. *Gann.* 1957; 48: 577-578.
28. Watanabe, T; Ibata, H; Sugikoto, T et al. Production and inhibition of hepatic sarcomata in rats by injections of trypan blue. *Gann.* 1957; 48: 576-577.
29. Evans, WH; Wolf, MM; Chabner, TA. Concentration of immature and mature granulocytes from normal human bone marrow. Proc. Soc. Exp. *Biol. Med.* 1974; 146:526-532.
30. Sokolov, II. About fusion of cellular nuclei. *Arch. Anat. Histol. Embryol.* 1955; 32: 54-62.
31. Tokoro, Y. Uber die artificielle erzeugung des sarkoms bei den weissen ratten mittels konzentrierte Kochsalzlosun. *Gann.* 1940; 34 :149-155.
32. Weisburger, JH; Weisburger, EK. Chemical substances as reason of cancer. *Usp. V. Izuchenii Raka.* 1969; VIII:501-539.

8 ONE AND THE SAME MECHANISM OF ACTION OF DIAMETRICALLY DIFFERENT CARCINOGENS

Transformation of normal cells into tumorous ones can be induced by the very different in their nature factors. Among them are numerous factors of physical (penetrating radiation of different nature), chemical (there are known more than 1500 carcinogenic chemical substances and combinations; regrettably, their number constantly increases) and biological nature (toxins of different kind, infectious and oncogenic viruses, etc.), what is confirmed by the data of experimental and clinical oncology and epidemiological analysis [1]. The same effect is induced by some pharmacological agents, oral contraceptives, irritations, burns, traumas, chronic inflammations and so on. A large number of carcinogens and the wide spectrum of their actions may indicate their ability to trigger a common, general mechanism inside the normal biological program of somatic cells, which can lead to the development of the carcinogenic transformation of the normal cell. Numerous carcinogenic substances and factors of different natures enumerated above probably can signify that these carcinogens must start up some common mechanism of normal cells transition into transformed states.

What are the common signs of all these above-mentioned factors, so different by their nature, as, for example, chemical substances, viruses, radiation of different kinds, glucose, plastics and so on? Is the mechanism of the cells' malignant transformation adequate to the influence of the very different carcinogenic and noncarcinogenic factors?

By our opinion the common mechanism of action of diametrically different carcinogens on target-cells is disintegration (destructions, perforations) of the plasmatic membrane (induction of the different size perforations) and consequently development of fusogeny – fusion of somatic cells, which is characteristics for any somatic cells and finally development of karyogamy. Among the processes in which the normal eukaryotic somatic cell-built programs participate during the body's vital activity, the following should be mentioned: mitosis, differentiation, interphase, phagocytosis, endomitosis, apoptosis, necrobiosis, adhesion, and, fusing. Whwn speaking about the biological essence of fusing, its possibility to create polyploidy in somatic cells like endomitosis) that intensifies resistance of a respective organ to negative environmental factors deserves mentioning. Regrettably, this necessary on the face of it for the organism process is associated with the risks of malignant transformation of the fusion-developed binuclear and polyploidy cells.

In the opinion of some scientists, especially of adherents of virus-genetic theory of carcinogenesis, it is hard to imagine that influence of cellular surface by different carcinogens may alter cells genome; moreover, that inherited character of malignant transformation supposed exactly the cellular henome alteration [2].

From the position of the karyogamic theory, the action of any carcinogen is not associated directly with gene apparatus of cells. Alteration of the cell's genome is induced indirectly; that is, after the somatic cells' fusion and arising of precancerous, tetraploid cell.

As it is known, somatic cells never interact. There is always some type of space (intercellular space) between them which is roughly 100-200 A. As a result each cell maintains its autonomy as an independent unit. As it is thought the balance between the attraction and reppulsion should be maintained at this 100-00 A interval. If for any reason the interval become less than 10 A, formation of Ca bridges is starting leading to the long-term adhesion of the cell. Intercellular contacts are predominantly determined by two main factors: Van der Vaals (positive taxis) and electrostatic (negative taxis) forces contributing to the formation of membrane electric potential. It seems that pores in the plasma membrane on the somatic cells formed by the action of the different physical, chemical and biological agents, substantially decrease the negative charge of the plasma membrane. In different terms this process (perforation) leads to the weaking on the electrostatic forces and enhancement of the Van der Vaals forces helping somatic cells to overcome intercellular forces and enter into contact with each other. In the case of prolonged contact adhesion process will start to develop [3].

Thus, influence of physical, chemical, and biological carcinogenic agents on cells probably are adequate. After their influence, cells' fusion originates as a result of cytoplasmic membranes perforations (or modifications), i.e. formation in plasma membranes pores, what induces alteration of summary superficial charge of cells' surface. Because of these, cells acquire ability to approach each other (adhesion), what in many cases may be a premise for fusion process. Thus, the initial target of carcinogenic agents is cells' plasma membrane, but not the genetic apparatus of cells.

Carcinogens' doses probably have the secondary importance in the origin of tumorous cells; moreover, the high doses of carcinogens of different natures (as we see above) can become the reason of the destruction and following elimination of the somatic cells and precancerous, initiated cells, as well.

In some cases, carcinogenic agents induce twice or even triple cytopathogenic action on somatic cells: oncogenic (by formation of dikaryons), but in some cases, they induce arising of polykaryocytes and cytolysis in somatic cells (for instance, in immunocompetent cells), which in some cases induce immune deficiency of various degrees [4-7]. It is possible that such different effects of carcinogens on cells depend on the size of the plasma membranes' pores. In the case of big-sized pores, irreversible changes and cytolysis take place. For instance, high electrostimulation and prolonged impulses lead to partial increasing of quantity of polynuclear cells, but further increase of stimulation induces cellular lysis. In low dose of electrostimulation dikaryons are observed most frequently, but polykaryocytes are revealed, too. The injection of small doses of Shope sarcoma virus in newborn rabbits led to tumorogenesis, as well as generalized fibromatosis. The inoculation of the same virus at larger doses resulted in the production of degenerative inflammatory or necrotic effects. Thus, practically all the agents and influences favoring cell's plasma membranes perforations, are regarded as the possible causes of the formation of malignant tumors.

Thus, at the first stage of carcinogenesis, i.e. at the stage of initiation, two (or more) normal somatic cells of one organ or tissue (so-called target-organ or tissue for some kind of the carcinogenic agents) at some favorable conditions may create dikaryons (hetero- or homokaryons), but in some cases nonviable polykaryocytes, i.e. multinuclear cells as well. Presumably, during the perforation of cellular membranes induced by different carcinogenic and non-carcinogenic factors, the total charge of plasma membranes changes, and the cells acquire the capability of closely approaching (adhesion), which frequently, especially upon coincidence of the perforated parts, may serve as a prerequisite to fusion. At this stage, together with multinuclear cellular structures, the binuclear - hetero- or homokaryons - carriers of high carcinogenic potency are formed. As a result of karyogamy, i.e. after synchronous mitosis or simple mechanical assembly of nuclei heterokaryons (or homokaryons) mononuclear hybrid precancerous cells developes, with tetraploid (or hypotetraploid) set of chromosomes on initial stage of hybridization. Received as a result of somatic hybridization, the hybrid synkaryon is an initiated, immortal, precancerous cell, which exists in macro organism indefinitely for a long time. At the initiated stage of its formation, a tumor synkaryon evidently possesses a tetraploid or hypotetraploid set of chromosomes. Further, in the processes of promotion and tumor progression, after the segregation of some chromosomes, tumorous cells with aneuploid or even hyperdiploid set of chromosomes may arise. In extremely rare cases, tumorous cells possess even diploid, hypodiploid or even hyperhaploid sets of chromosomes.

On the promotion stage, after the influence of complete (perfect, full) carcinogens or promoters on tissue, where precancerous synkaryons preexist, in these cells the chromosomal aberrations of different types and genes amplifications may arise. One of the conditions in formation of both precancerous and tumorous cells are quantitative (tetraploid, subtetraploid, hyperdiploid, aneuploid and other types of sets of chromosomes) aberrations of chromosomes. The important attending process of cells' malignant conversion on promotion stage is hyperplasia, i.e. intensive proliferation of cells of the tissue, in which the precancerous synkaryon preexist. In the overwhelming majority of cases, because of unsuccessful mitosis (so-called lethal mitosis), elimination, perish of precancerous synkaryons probably takes place at stage of transformation into tumor synkaryons. However in rare cases, in result of specific (reciprocal or nonbalanced) translocations, duplications and following genes' amplifications, these cells may undergo irreversible alterations and may transform into true tumor cells (synkaryons of stage II).

From the chromosomal aberrations, the most dangerous in carcinogenic respect are nonbalanced translocations, and also duplications, expressed in "complementation" of chromosomes' identical sites, having the same function. This event usually leads to genes' amplification, in consequence of which expression of genes (oncogenes), responsible for the control under the cellular proliferation, ultimately may originate.

In the process of tumor progression, segregation of some chromosomes in the tumorous synkaryon, and also involvement last cells by means of fusion of considerably amount of other cancerous cells and normal cells of different types and maturity take place. After this tumorous cells with extreme polymorphism of karyotype and new abilities, arise. Notwithstanding the fact that a tumor substrate originates initially from one synkaryon, or despite its clonal character, in most cases, the tumorous cells of higly morphologic and cytogenetic polymorphism originate. Cellular subpopulations are constantly formed in them tumor focus without any obvious regularity and can coexist in the phenotypically and genotypically distinguished cells.

Thus, malignant tumors have clonal origin and on initial stage consist of genetically identical cells. In the future, cellular tumor substrate develops continuously and alters genetic properties. As it was shown, in most cases, malignant neoplasms in late stages of carcinogenesis (progression) are heterogenic in antigen composition, as by metastatic abilities, by character of growth on plastic substrate, and in cytogenetic, ultrastructure and histochemical signs as well [8-10]. The karyogamic theory of carcinogenesis (or the theory of "two synkaryons") explaines these facts by the spontaneous or induced somatic hybridization of tumor cells, or tumor and precancerous cells, or of tumor and normal cells of the tumor substrate.

Thus, it could be concluded that physical, chemical, and biological carcinogens and influences lead to similar result: to induction of cells malignization by means of somatic hybridization. Consequently, hybridization of somatic cells represents itself as one of the possible mechanism of malignant conversion. The formed as a result of this process heterokaryons, homokaryons and synkaryons should be considered as the basis (substratum) of malignant growth. It may be also concluded that the malignant growth is a polyetiologic and concurrently a monopathogenetic process.

At the same time, in distinction from the generally accepted modern views in oncology, which consider, that initiated agents influence the cells' genotype (genotropic, genotoxic actions), by the karyogamic theory of carcinogenesis, initiated agents in the first instance interact with the cells' plasma membranes, inducing their perforations, fusion process and only then cells' somatic hybridization (i.e. quantitative aberrations of chromosomes) [11-14].

Here we are trying to answer one of the most complex questions in oncology from the view of karyogamic theory: are the chromosomal aberrations the cause or the consequence of the cancerous growth? We hypothesize that during initiation (formation of precancerous cells) chromosomal aberrations (quantitative aberrations) are on the third place after the perforations of the plasmatic membrane and fusogeny (formation of dikaryons). During promotion (i.e. formation of true cancerous cells) chromosomal aberrations (first of all structural aberrations) are on the first place before the gene amplification. In the case of progression (formation of cancerous cells with a new genotypes and phenotypes) the sequence should be the same as for the initiation (perforations, fusogeny and after that - chromosomal aberrations). So the role of chromosomal aberrations differs at the different stages of carcinogenesis, but there are no doubts about their causative connections: at the stages of initiation and progression (invasion) chromosomal aberrations are among the main causative factors. After the plasmatic membrane perforations, this organoids electric charge decrease. In result of this, formed dikaryons, what is in some cases prerequisite of fusogeny. At the stage of promotion, the main causative factor is the structural chromosomal aberrations [15].

Thus, chromosomal aberrations (as quantitative, as structural) are one of the direct reasons of tumorous process, but not its consequence. These chromosomal aberrations originated only after fusion of somatic cells, in particular, from a moment of precancerous cell arising; i.e., on initial phase take place perforations of cell's plasma membranes by carcinogenic agents, then, change of the electric charge, arising of dikaryons (hetero- and homokaryons), and only an moment of arising of precancerous cell (synkaryon of stage I), begin of genetical processes involving. After the above conversion on the subcellular and molecular levels, there may arise a true tumor synkaryon (so-called synkaryon of stage II), malignant cell with the ability of uncontrolled proliferation. The synkaryon of stage II represents the clone, from which formation of malignant tumors substrate at the early stage of carcinogenesis begins.

CONCLUSION

The common mechanism of action of diametrically different carcinogens is the disintegration (perforation) of the plasmatic membrane and consequently development of fusogeny and finally, of karyogamy. Thus, influence of different carcinogenic agents on cells is adequate. Formation in plasma membranes perforations induces alteration of summary superficial charge of cells' surface. Because of these, somatic cells acquire ability to approach each other, what in many cases may be a premise for fusion process.

REFERENCES

1. Cohen, SM; Arnold, LL. Chemical carcinogenesis. *Toxicological Sciences*. 2011; 120 (suppl.1):576-592.
2. Zilber, LA. *Virus-genetic theory of tumor formation*. Moscow. 1968.
3. Minuk, GY; Zhang, M; Gong, Y. et al. Decreased hepatocyte membrane potential differences and BABAa-B3 expression in human hepatocellular carcinoma. *Hepatology*. 2007; 45:735-745.
4. Vaananen, P; Kaarianen, L. Fusion and hemolysis of erythrocytes caused by three togaviruses: Semliki Forest, Sindbis and Rubella. *J.Gen.Virol*. 1980; 46:467-475.
5. Huang, RT; Rott,R; Klenk,HD. Influenza viruses cause haemolysis and fusion of cells. *Virology*.1981; 110:243-247.
6. White, G; Metlin, K; Helenius, A. Cell fusion by Semliki Forest, influenza, and vesicular stomatitis viruses. *J.Cell Biol*. 1981; 89: 674-679.
7. Owens, RJ, Burke, C, Rose, JK. Mutations in the membrane-spanding domain of the human immunodeficiency virus envelope glycoprotein that affect fusion activity. *J. Virol*. 1994; 68:570-574.
8. Nowell, PS. The clonal evolution of tumor cell population. *Science*. 1976; 194:23-28.
9. Woodruff, MFA. What's going on in the cancer patient? *Pathology*. 1986; 18:175-180.
10. Leder, LD. Zur individualitat von malignen neoplasien. *Strahlanther und Oncol.*. 1986; 162:624-628.
11. Gogichadze, G; Misabishvili, E; Gogichadze, T. Tumor cell formation by normal somatic cells fusing and cancer prevention prospects. *Med. Hypotheses*. 2006; 66 :133-136.

12. Gogichadze, G; Gogichadze, T. *Karyogamic theory of cancer cell formation from the view of the XXI century.* Nova Biomedical Books, New York. 2010.
13. Gogichadze G. Common characteristics of a cancer cell and logical corroborations of its hybrid essence. *Advances in Genetic Research. Ed. Kevin V. Urbano. Nova Science Publishers, Inc. New York.* 2011; 46:161-178.
14. Gogichadze, GK; Gogichadze, TG. *Somatic hybridization, as a primary reason of malignization.* Lambert Academic Publisher, Saarbruken, 2013.
15. Wolman, SR. Cytogenetic heterogeneity: its role in tumor evolution. *Cancer Genet.Cytogenet.* 1986, 19:129-140.

    Gogichadze GK. Gogichadze T., Kamkamidze G. Presumably Common Trigger Mechanism of Action of Diametrically Different Carcinogens on Target Cells. Cancer and Oncology Research, 2013, 1 (2), p.65-68.

9 INITIATORS, PROMOTERS AND COMPLETE CARCINOGENS FROM STANDPOINT OF KARYOGAMIC THEORY

Malignant conversion of the somatic cells into tumor ones can be assisted by the very different in their nature agents and factors: penetrating radiation of different nature, chemical carcinogens, some oncogenic and infectious viruses, some pharmacological agents, biotoxins, for instance, mycotoxins, snake venom and so on), some kinds of irritations, etc. Thus, transformation of normal cells into tumor ones can be induced by the very different in their nature agents and factors, what is confirmed by the data of experimental and clinical oncology and epidemiological analyses.

A special carcinogenic danger represents weak or middle doses of radiation and chemical substances. Majority of tumors are characterized by the increase of frequency of their formations with increase of irradiation dose to a definite level and reduction of frequency of tumors when exceeding this level of irradiation. Probably, above-enumerated carcinogens start up some a common mechanism of the conversion of normal cells into transformated state.

A plurality of factors promoting induction of the malignant growth considerably reduces the hope of tumors monoetiogenesis and proceeding from this, on elaboration of etiotropic treatment of this fatal disease. Numerous carcinogenic substances and factors of different nature must start up some common mechanism of normal cells transition into tumor one.

What are the common signs of all these above-mentioned factors, so different by their nature, as, for example chemical substances, oncogenic and infection viruses, radiation of different kind, glucose, plastics and so on? Is the mechanism of cells malignant transformation adequate to the influence of the very different carcinogenic and noncarcinogenic factors? (In more detail see Chapter 8).

Firstly it is necessary to emphasize that some of above-mentioned agents and factors can possess as initiating, so promoter's qualities. Thus, they are complete or full carcinogens. Complete carcinogens induces tumors without the additional influence of the other agents and factors. Other agents influence the cells only as initiators or promoters. Later agents by themselves can not induce malignant tumors. In other words, if in experimental animals, after action of any carcinogens tumors are formed, which are not observed in control series, one may conclude that this substance induced tumors de novo and consequently represented complete (full) carcinogen. If after action of this or another substance spontaneous tumors become only more frequent, this substance is called as incomplete carcinogen or promoter.

From the hybridization theory of the origin of malignant neoplasms we can suppose that complete (full, perfect) carcinogenic substances and factors (also initiators) create in the organism such a condition, when formation of precancerous cells is possible; in particular, they influence cellular membranes, induce in them perforations (pores of different size), stimulating process of somatic hybridization and subsequently possibility of precancerous cells formation. At the same time, promoting factors (promoters and complete carcinogens) assist in stimulating proliferative activity of already formed after the influence of carcinogens, initiated, i.e. precancerous cells, transforming them into tumorous ones. As known, promoters induce inflammation processes in skin, hyperplastic changes in epidermis, etc.

Many above enumerated carcinogenic factors have specific effect on definite organs and tissue of macro organism (so-calles critical or target organs). Example of such tropism can be: cancer of scrotum in the case of chimney-sweep's, lympho- and monoblastic sarcomas in transplantations of allogenic internal organs, chronic myeloleukaemias in the most cases of malignant tumors after exposition to atomic explosions in Hiroshima and Nagasaki and so on. In connection with the last observations, hemopoietic system, especially myeloid stem of bone marrow becomes most vulnerable to radiation of this kind. According to the available data, the first in the group of malignant diseases, striking the population as a result of radiation, are leukaemias of different forms, but on the following (more remote) places are cancer of mammary and thyroid glands, lung cancer, lymphomas of different types and so on.

The concept that the transformation of normal cells into tumor ones is not a simple, single-stage mutated process but rather a multistage progressive act has been essentially confirmed recently. Neverthless, the same idea was surmised to the middle XX century by P.Rous and J.Kidd [1]. These scientists supposed that malignant neoplasms may develop from one cell, which in the malignization process may involve two or more stages.

The terms "initiation" and "promotion" were first suggested by W.Friedewald and P.Rous in 1944 [2]. In 1947, I.Berenblum and P.Scubik developed in more detail the concept of two-stage mechanism of carcinogenesis [3]. Following this concept, we may assume that during the initiation process, there occurs a transformation of normal cells into a latent, precancerous cell, the growth and propagation of which is not realized by the corresponding control systems of the organism.

The lengthy latent period of some carcinogenic agents is supposedly a result of a two-stage or multistage malignization process [4]. The transformation of initiated cell into a true tumor one may take place only occasionally, without an essential latent period (for example, under the influence of so-called short-lived carcinogens, such as nitrosamides or during a prolonged action on the organism of complete carcinogens or under a synergic action of different carcinogens).

It has long been established that the application in animals first of promoters and only later of carcinogens does not trigger tumor growth. An interval between the effect of carcinogen and beginning of promoters' (for instance, croton oil) exposition may be many months, without a significant reduction of the carcinogenic effect. The promoter's action is slow, gradual; therefore, its effect on the target tissue should be lengthy. A suspension of the promoter's action will lead to regress of the carcinogenic process.

According to modern concepts, initiation is induced by the so-call initiators and complete carcinogens and may be irreversible stage. Formed as a result of initiation, precancerous (latent, initialized, immortalized) cells possess an altered genotype. As regards promotion, the process may be carried out by the so-called promoters (i.e., non-carcinogenic factors), complete carcinogens, and may be reversible stage. Presumably, a prolonged proliferation of cells stimulated by different causes (complete carcinogens, promoters, etc.) facilitates the forming of tumor synkaryon. Cells being in a stage of division secrete substances (the growth factor) that stimulate the process of mitosis of other cells (for instance, precancerous cells). In other words, hyperplasia, i.e. an intensive proliferation of respective tissue cells, is an prerequisite for realizing the oncogenic potentials of definite carcinogenic and non-carcinogenic factors and effects. Moreover, tumorous often exist in tissues whose cells sometimes divide and are actually absent in the tissues where cells generally do not divide or divide rarely.

Irrespective of an intensive study of the carcinogenesis initiation and promotion stages, details and specific mechanisms of the action of initiators, promoters and complete carcinogens on the target cells and tissues have not been sufficiently understood. Below, we give a comprehensive (in our opinion) definition of initiators, promoters and complete carcinogens and the presumable mechanisms of their action on target cells from the standpoint of the karyogamic theory of carcinogenesis.

1. According to the karyogamic theory of carcinogenesis, as a result of the mechanism of fusogeny (or fusion of normal somatic cells) initiators and complete carcinogens form at the initial stage of oncogenesis first a dikaryon and then, as a result of karyogamy (synchronous mitosis and/or mechanical fusion of cells nuclei) – a hybrid, mononuclear synkaryon, the same precancerous cell [5-9]. As it seems, even in the case of a single action of a small dose of complete carcinogen or initiator at the initial stage, the initiating situation occurs or the formation of a precancerous cell (synkaryon of stage I) takes place in the respective tissue. Such a cell has an altered genotype (tetraploid or hypotetraploid set of chromosomes at the initial stage), while its phenotype is mostly unaltered.

Thus, *initiator* is the agent that causes development of the initial stage of carcinogenesis (in other words, formation of the precancerous cell) but cannot form a tumor cell without a promoter. Its single action on the respective tissue (or cell) is sufficient for developing the initiating process. Seemingly, the initiator interacts directly with plasma membrane rather than with the cell genome. According to the karyogamic theory of carcinogenesis, any agent or factor causing the plasma membrane perforation can be regarded as a carcinogenic potential carrier, i.e. the initiator or even the complete carcinogen. It should be mentioned here that it is doubtful whether complete or pure initiators exist or whether a part of them possesses carcinogenic properties as well. Some viruses, fatty acids, carbohydrates, etc. can be named as initiators of carcinogenesis. Based on the fact that the virus provokes the formation of a precancerous rather than malignant cell, it can be concluded that the carcinogenesis process initiator should be a virus rather than a complete carcinogen.

2. *Promoter* is the agent which provokes the transfer of a precancerous cell already formed as a result of initiation stagel. It is associated with such processes as the amplification of genes, the aberration of chromosomes, also the inflammatory changes in the respective tissue or organ (for example, skin), hyperplasia of the target cell (e.g. epidermis), etc. At this stage, following an inbalances or reciprocal (which is less expected) translocation (or chromosomal aberrations of other type) and gene amplification, the precancerous cell may undergo an irreversible change and transform into a true tumor cell. Generally, the induction of proliferation is a promoter's concomitant property. It is unknown whether there exist complete (pure) promoters, especially as a part of them was found to have although weak but still carcinogenic properties. An interval between the complete carcinogen and promoter action can take several months, without a significant reduction of the carcinogenic effect. One of the most known

promoters is the croton oil. The role of a promoter can also be assumed by saccharin, Tween 60, DDT, phenobarbital, trauma, etc. Study of promoters is of importance not only for understanding the mechanism of carcinogenesis, but also in practical terms: substances with promoting properties are used for preparing drugs, food additives, etc..

In parallel with the structural aberrations of chromosomes in a tumor cell (synkaryon of stage II) at the stage of promotion, a quantitative instability of chromosomes takes place. One of the causes of the above is a definite segregation of chromosomes leading to quantitative changes in the cell: frequently, tetraploidy can be substituted with hypotetraploidy, hyperdiploidy, etc. Most important is that a tumor cell could preserve such a number of chromosomes that would enable a successful implementation of mitosis. In other, much frequent cases, the lethal or imbalanced mitosis will take place and ultimately lead to the cell loss. Another cause of the chromosomal instability in a tumor cell consists in a facilitated fusogeny of cancer cells with the cells of other type. For example, in the process of tumor progression, the segregation of some chromosomes in a cancer synkaryon and fusion with a considerable number of other tumor cells and normal cells of different type and maturity take place. As a result, tumor cells with extreme polymorphism of karyotype and new abilities arise.

3. Complete carcinogen provokes the development of tumors without any additional action, i.e. it is known for both the initiating and promotion activity. Thus, complete carcinogens can provoke perforations of the target cell's plasma membranes (as initiators), as well as the proliferating activity of the respective tissue (as promoters). To the number of complete carcinogens can be included: radiation of different type, benzpyrene, vinyl chloride, pesticides, toxins, some viruses, etc.

CONCLUSION

According to the karyogamic theory of carcinogenesis, any agent causing the plasma membrane perforation can be regarded as a carcinogenic potential carrier, i.e. the initiator or even the complete carcinogen. Promoter provokes the transformation of a precancerous cell already formed as a result of initiation process. Complete carcinogen provokes the development of tumors without any additional action, i.e. it is known for both the initiating and promotion activity.

REFERENCES

1. Rous, P; Kidd, J. Conditional neoplasms and subthreshold neoplastic states. *J.Exptl.Med.* 1941; 73:365-372.
2. Friedewald, WF; Rous, P. The initiating and promoting elements in tumor production: an analysis of the effects of tar, berzpyrene, and methylcholanthrene on rabbit skin. *J.Exp.Med.* 1944; 8:101-126.
3. Berenblum, I; Scubik, P. A new quantitative approach to the study of the stages of chemical carcinogenesis in the mous's skin. *Brit.J.Cancer.* 1947; 1:383-390
4. Van Den Hoof, A. The enigmatic role of asbestos in malignancies the lung. *Anticancer Res.* 1986; 6:199-201.
5. Hallion, L. Sur la pathogenie du cancer; theorie karyogamique. *Press Med. Par.* 1907; XV:10-11.
6. Gogichadze, GK. Possible role of somatic hybridization in mechanism of a malignant transformation of cells. *Hematol. Transfusiol.* 1989; 6:54-57.
7. Gogichadze, GK. Common characteristics of cancer cell and logical corroborations of its hybrid essence. *Advances in Genetic Research. Ed. K.Urbano. Nova Science Publishers, Inc. New York.* 2011; 46: 161-178.
8. Gogichadze, GK; Misabishvili, EV; Gogichadze, TG. Tumor cells formation by normal somatic cells fusing and cancer prevention prospects. *Med. Hypotheses.* 2006; 66:133-136.
9. Gogichadze, GK; Gogichadze, TG. *Karyogamic theory of cancer cell formation from the view of the XXI century.* Nova Biomedical Books, New York. 2010.

10 MOLECULAR GENETIC ASPECTS OF CARCINOGENESIS AT ITS DIFFERENT STEPS

Among the hypotheses and theories dedicated to the problem of carcinogenesis, karyogamic theory belongs to those rare theories which deal with both etiology and pathogenesis of cancer formation [1]. This theory maybe considered as general (common or integrate) theory of carcinogenesis, which includes the principal aspects of the most popular and acceptable theories and hypotheses for today [2,3]. Based on this theory it was suggested that Influence of diametrically different carcinogens on target cells probably are adequate. After their influence, cells' fusion originates as a result of cytoplasmic membranes perforations [4]. It would be interesting to discuss details of the genetic aspects related with each stage of the carcinogenesis (initiation, promotion and progression).

10.1 Initiation

Polypotent cells or other commited cells sensitive to carcinogenic effects and capable of proliferation form firstly dikaryons (hetero- or homokaryons) and than hybrid cells (synkaryons) by means of fusion with another cells of the same organism, in particular, with differentiated and non-differentiated cells of corresponding tissue or with cells capable to migrate (macrophages, granulocytes of different maturity and so on).

In all probability, during the perforation or modification of the plasma membrane, i.e., after the formation of pores, induced by different carcinogenic agents and factors, the total charge of this organoid changes and cells develop the ability to come closer to each other, which frequently, especially upon coincidence of the perforated parts, will probably be the prerequisite to a fusion process [5].

In the opinion of adherents of the virus-genetic theory of carcinogenesis, it is hard to imagine that influence of cellular surface by carcinogens may alter cells' genome; moreover, that inherited character of malignant transformation supposed exactly the cellular genome alteration. From the position of the karyogamic theory of carcinogenesis, the action of any carcinogen is not associated directly with gene apparatus of cells. Alteration of the cell's genome is induced indirectly.

It is necessary to emphasize that in most cases, dikaryons (hetero- or homokaryons) probably perish in this stage as a result of lethal fusion (karyogamy) of nuclei. On the other hand, after successful karyogamy of nuclei mononuclear synkaryon is formed, which is differ from normal parent cells genotypically and possess on the early stage tetraploid or hypotetraploid sets of chromosomes. Fusion immediately doubles the number of chromosomes, thereby decreasing the chances that the loss of some chromosomes will kill the hybrid cell. In synkaryon, formed on the following stages of development, the segregation, i.e., elimination of definite chromosomes, is possible. More often, in precancerous cells, an assumptive set of chromosomes must be hypotetraploid or hyperdiploid one.

A chromosomal combinations of different types (tetraploidy, aneuploidy) is lethal and, as a result, the creation of such hybrids do not effect the development of the macro organism and the entire species. Any anomaly of the karyotype has no negative effect on the body, provided the cell with such karyotype cannot divide and initiate the autonomous evolution.

Precancerous (initiated, immortal) cells-synkaryons in phenotypic respect, in most cases, are almost indistinguishable from normal cells of these tissue, as they retain morphology similar to the one of the parent cells. Only in rare cases, because of intermediate heredity, precancerous cells may have morphology of the both parent cells simultaneously, i.e., intermediate morphology. These synkaryons differ from normal cells only by their genotype, having tetraploid chromosome set at the initial stage of fusion, and then hypotetraploid, hyperdiploid set of chromosomes and so on. Precancerous cells, can be remained in the organism in latent state for indefinite by long time, probably in some cases for decades.

Taking into consideration the plurality and variety of environmental carcinogenic agents and factors around us, and also the fact the the polypotent cells, stem cells, lymphocytes, macrophages and commited cells exist in all tissue of macro organism, one can suppose that precancerous cells can often be formed in many tissue and organs simultaneously. Thus, theoretically, we can expect that in all tissue of one organism can be simultaneously accumulated precancerous cells. For example, there are communications about simultaneosly developed tumors of different localization and histogenesis [6].

Thus, on initiation stage of carcinogenesis, normal somatic cells form dikaryons, carriers of high carcinogenic potency, and giant polykaryocytes. These last cells in most cases, are nonviable cellular formation, i.e., in the genetic respect, they probably are defective peculiar forms, with the lost abilities to enter in S-period of cellular cycle and mitosis. Giant polykaryocytes, in the whole, must be interpreted solely as a reactive process, carried out in all tissues and organs of macro organism at pathologic states. Thus, it is necessary to take into consideration that the appearance in certain tissues and organs of polykaryocytes can signify presence of conditions for cells' hybridization and, consequently, potential possibility of appearance of tumorous dikaryons and then synkaryons.

10.2 Promotion

The mechanism of malignant transformation of the precancerous cell into a tumorous one probably has the molecular and sub-cellular foundations.

For tumor promotion (i.e., formation of tumorous synkaryon) the necessary precondition is active proliferation (hyperplasia) of the corresponding tissue. In the process of promotion, i.e., under the effect of perfect carcinogens, promoters, non-specific influences or some extreme situations (fractures, traumas, and resections) stimulating carcinogenesis, a precancerous synkaryon can transform into a tumorous synkaryon. Prolonged proliferation of cells caused by various reasons is one of the major conditions, during which the carcinogenic potency of different substances and factors fully manifests itself.

Thus, in the process of promotion, a precancerous synkaryon can be transformed into tumorous one. The mechanism of malignant transformation probably has the molecular and sub-cellular conditions. Some sites of certain chromosomes seem to have a great significance for the control of the intensity of cell's proliferation and differentiation. In rare cases, as a result of specific chromosome translocation or other chromosome aberrations, which may lead to the amplification of genes, controlling the intensity of proliferation, the so-called "over-expressed gene" can be formed [7]. It is necessary to emphasize that in resemblance with diploid cells, in cells with tetraploid (likely, with hypotetraploid or hyperdiploid and so on) set of chromosomes clearly tend to formation of chromosomes' aberrations. Over-expressed genes may function permanently, coding so-called cancer albumen (or the "growth factor") in great amounts, then suffer anomaly activity of cell, which is characteristic for malignant state. In this case, the precancerous cell acquired the ability of intensive and uncontrolled proliferation. These cells may pass into the stage of promotion, i.e., they transforms into true tumorous synkaryon. This last cell acquires selective advantage over the normal cells.

As known, complete carcinogens and initiators can induce damage on level on genes. Such damages are: gene amplification, protooncogene activation, violations of DNA physiological methylation and so on. Violations can be brought on chromosomal level as well. Such alterations are chromosomes structural aberrations, such as translocations (reciprocal and nonbalanced), deletions, duplications, inversions. Chromosome number alterations (heteroploidy), ultimately make conditions for aneuploidy of a chromosome set, attribute loss or addition of separate chromosomes (or locus of chromosomes), what takes place as a result of their incorrect divergences in mitosis [8,9].

In a process of promotion, i.e., influence of carcinogens, promoters or modifying factors, which stimulate proliferation of somatic cells, precancerous cell, in some rare cases, as a result of chromosomal translocations or of other types of chromosomal aberrations, what, for its part, can lead to genes amplification, can be transformed into tumorous synkaryon.

Thus, structural alterations, i.e., aberrations of chromosomes, usually lead to the loss (deletion) or acquisition of individual sites of chromosomes, i.e., to nonbalanced or reciprocal translocations and duplications. Transferring of part of genetical material from one chromosome to another, ultimately, can lead to the alterations in expression of definite genes. It is necessary to mark that the transfer of genetic material from one chromosome to another occurs not only in translocations, but in other types of chromosomes' aberrations, too. For instance, in duplication of one chromosome, or in different nonhomological chromosomes, analogous sites of chromosomes (in several specimens) are present, having the same function. Duplicated sites in chromosomes frequently form the tandem, i.e., they are located one after another. As to deletion, this type of chromosome aberration in some cases may also participate in gene's activation, but, of course, not by amplification of one or another oncogene. In the case of deletion, as it is known, the loss of genetic material is observed, which can lead to the expression of the oncogene, which was controlled (e.g., repressed) by the lost chromosome site.

Thus, in the mechanism of oncogenes' activation, different structural aberrations of chromosomes (translocations, duplications and possibly deletions) can take part. However, the majority of researchers put the main accent on chromosomes' specific translocation, as on reciprocal, as well as especially on nonbalanced translocations.

It is probable, that gene amplification is one of the possible mechanisms of cellular oncogene activation, what can lead to undesirable gene's expression resulting in abnormal proliferative activity of precancerous cells.

The actual existence of the above-mentioned molecular (sub-cellular) mechanism of normal somatic cells' transformation has been confirmed by recent studies, which establish that various carcinogenic factors and influences are the inductors of genes' amplification [10,11].

Theoretically, even a single amplification of corresponding genes by any dose of promoters is a sufficient condition for conversion of normal cells into malignant state.

Tumorous cells formed by means of above mechanism, because of expression or the increase of dose of genes, are distinguished by their ability to more intensive proliferation, what gives selective advantage as compared with the normal cells. After one cellular division, such cell may get over the rails of progression.

Why are the oncogenic diseases comparatively rare? Given that cancer by its prevalence shares the first and second positions with cardiovascular diseases, while the statistical analysis indicates its rather high frequency (40-100 new cancer cases per 100,000 men, or 80 cases on average, i.e. 0,08%), account should be taken of the following circumstances: 1.What does the concept "prevalent" mean? It would, naturally, be good if no case of cancer was recorded per 100,000 men, but still … what is "prevalent"? Are 40-120 cases prevalent and 30-35 are not? 2.Notwithstanding prevalence and irreversibility of the initiation stage and that under the karyogamic theory precancerous cells exist in any organ and tissue of a macro organism and in spite of the fact that the fusogeny process, together with phagocytosis mitosis, meiosis and other processes, is genetically included in any somatic cell development program, the genuine malignant cell's origination is luckily is still rather rare.

On the one hand, taking into consideration the environment of human external carcinogenic background and plurality of complete carcinogens and also initiators (number of which increases permanently), one can make assumptions about the frequent origin of precancerous cells. On the other hand, at promotion, to transform precancerous cells into tumorous ones, some coincidences on the molecular and sub-cellular levels are necessary (nonbalanced treanslocation or other chromosomal aberrations, genes' amplifications). Out of the numerous dikaryons and synkaryons formed after the influence of carcinogenic agents, only a few precancerous cells can acquire the potency of unlimited proliferation. In the overwhelming majority of cases, they seem to die in the phase of transformation into tumorous cells due to lethal mitosis. Specifically, because of the imbalance of karyotypes, they either never reach mitosis or are unable to complete it due to disturbance in spindle organization or chromosomes motion. Therefore, true tumorous synkaryons are probably formed very rarely. Only one out of a million of precancerous cells has the prospects of conversion into a geneuine cancer cell.

If it were not for the so high percentage of lethal mitosis during karyogamy and particularly upon transformation of precancerous cells into a genuine cancer cell, the existence of the civilization proper would be endangered and the researchers claiming that cancer might be the last stage of the human ontogenesis would appear to be correct.

10.3 Progression

Any combinations of cancer cell with other differentiated and nondifferentiated normal somatic cells are possible. This is the reason for different histogenesis and heterogeneity (morphologic, cytogenetic, antigenic and, etc.) of tumorous cells. Thus, the population of tumorous cells, as morphologically, as cytogenetically (and on other signs) in spite of clonal origin of tumors, often is highly heterogenous. Cellular subpopulations are constantly formed in tumors without any obvious regularity and in any other tumor can coexist there phenotypically and genotypically different cells.

In the case of progression, generalization of tumor process, exacerbation, a transition to a more malignant stage take place. The progression stage, as it seems, should be conditioned by two radically different from one another properties of a tumor cells, which is being manifested in the ability to develop invasion process, in the one case, and the metastatic process, in the other case. These two processes, i.e. invasion and metastasis, significantly differ from one another by their development, cellular mechanisms, etc. In particular, in the invasion process, inclusion by tumor cells of the neighbour new normal somatic cells in the fusion process takes place, as a result of which tumor cells of new phenotype and genotype are formed. In contrast to it, in the metastasis process, the development of secondary tumors in a macro organism takes place, as a result of breaking-away of some cells from the initial tumor. In the case of invasion and metastasis, a great importance in seemingly given to a changeable electric charge value. However, if in the case of metastasis the electric charge on the tumor cell's surface counts during almost the whole process, in the case of invasion such charge will count only upon a contact between a tumor cell and its neighbour normal somatic cell, which enables the convergence and further adhesion of these cells.

10.3.1 Invasion

Separate clones of specific malignant tumors can differ from each other in many abilities, including their metastatic potency, antigen composition, sensitivity to different factors and influences and so on. The origin of clonal divergence may be the consequence of genetic instability of tumorous cells, what unlimitely leads to the tumor progression. The genetic mechanism of tumor progression and tumorous cells heterogeneity is so far vague and possibly depends on complicated interrelation between the macro organism and the tumor.

We can make the assumption that the possible mechanism of morphological, cytogenetical, etc., heterogeneities of cancer cells and tumor invasion consist in the further involuntary somatic hybridization of these cells. Moreover, it may be possible that in tumorous cells, in resemblance with normal ones, the ability for somatic hybridization is abnormally high.

We suppose that the process of invasion is taking place when the tumor tissue's pH is low. Notwithstanding the fact that progression is the final stage of carcinogenesis (following initiation and promotion stages), and the invasion is one of the characteristic properties of the cancer cell, we think that it would not be a great mistake if we temporarily combine the both notions, especially as they appear to have almost the same mechanism: in particular, it should include the involvement by the cancer cells of new cellular partners first in the process of fusion and then hybridization.

It the known fact that cancer cells, as compared with normal analogs, much easier enter the hybridization process with other normal cells. If we rationate, in the presence of a high negative charge cancer cells should not have the ability to effect somatic hybridization with other cells with such intensity. Apparently, invasion should occur only in the case when cancer cells have a low negative, neutral or even a positive charge. Concurrently, the prerequisite for fusiong of cells are perforations of the plasma membrane of both cellular partners (cancer cell and other cancer cell, cancer cell and precancerous cell or normal cell). In case the plasma membranes of these cells lack pores (holes), these cells will contact with each other but without fusing. The same result is expected in the case of availability of pores in the plasma membrane of one cellular partner only.

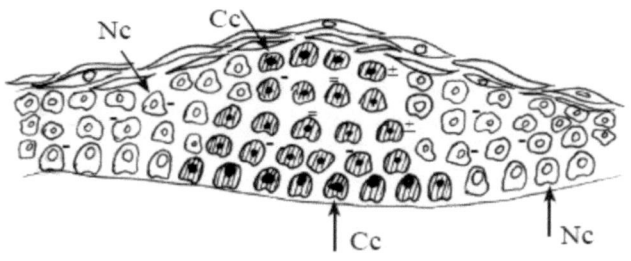

Fig. 2. Invasion
Abbreviations: Cc – cancer cells; Nc – normal cells;
- - negative charge; ± - neutral charge;
= - high negative charge.

On the other hand, the active cell metabolism has been found to condition the suppression of pH towards the acid medium. In its turn, the acid medium contributes to the formation of pores (holes) in the plasma membranes of cells, this being accompanied with the negative electric charge suppression on the cell surface. This circumstance is contributive to cell-to cell-contacts, further adhesion and fusing. Moreover that the possibility of the formation of dikaryons or symplast-like structures during low pH is a long-established fact (see Chapter 5). Thus, in the case of low pH it is quite possible that the formation of pores on plasma membranes of both partner cells, adhesion, the formation of dikaryons, then karyogamy and, as a result, the process of invasion can take place. In the case of inmvasion, further genotypic and phenotypic changes are taking place.

Thus, it may be supposed that a possible mechanism of invasion process is the hybridization of somatic cells, i.e., the already formed tumorous cells can be often hybridized both with the same cells and with normal cells [12]. After the fusion with other tumorous cells or with normal cellular elements, formation of dikaryons may take place, in which one nucleus can be represented by tumorous cells, and the second, by normal cells (in case of fusion of tumor and normal cells). After synchronous mitosis or mechanical assembly of nuclei in such cells, a hybrid cell-synkaryon can be formed. This cellular type is represented with new genotypic (and in some cases phenotypic, as well) signs.

10.3.2 Metastasis

To understand the mechanisms responsible for metastasis is one of the priority goals of cancer research. This process remains one of the most enigmatic aspects of this fatal disease.

Only some cells of the primary cancer are able to metastize (the ability of breaking off from the main focus, migration and attachment to a new place). Once the cancer cell is detached from the primary tumor, it will penetrate blood vessels (or lymphatic chanels), retaining viability under the damaging and lethal to it influence, such as blood turbulence and contacts with the immune system cells. Further, by passing the basement membrane, it will go from the blood-vessel endothelium to the target organ. Thus, in order to initiate the process of metastasis, the cancer cell must get detached from the primary tumor seat and penetrate the basement membrane twice in two different directions – from the tumor seat to blood vessels (capillary) and then from the blood vessels to the target organ's tissue. In order to perform such a complex migration, it is necessary that essential alterations of electric potential on the plasma membrane of the cancer cell take place, which should be associated with the hydrogenous index (pH) changes.

The membrane potential of a cancer cell plasmalemma should be connected with the changes of physical and chemical nature occuring in the macro organism, as well as with the metabolic activity of this type of cells proper. The cancer cell metabolism has been found to differ from the normal cell metabolism. Cancer cells can switch on and activated alternative biochemical processes, enhancing thus the metabolism of these cells. As a result, the environmental pH is suppressed. In the case of a relatively suppressed metabolism of cancer cells, the environmental pH increases. In the case of high pH, a cancer cell may develop a high negative charge, which suppresses its adhesion with the tumor bulk and can lead to its detachment and migration in the macro organism. In the event of enhanced metabolism of a cancer cell, the environmental pH is suppressed, as a result of which cancer cells acquire a relatively low negative, neutral or even a positive charge on their surface. Should a metastatic cell change its high negative charge for a relatively low negative, neutral or even a positive charge, its attachment to a new place and the formation of new cancer cell populations will be quite real. In contrast to metastasis, invasion process should take place only if cancer cells have a low negative, neutral or positive charge [13].

Overall, the process of metastasis can, as it seems, be diveded into 6 stages: 1) the growth of a new network of blood vessels, called tumor angiogenesis; 2) the metastatic cell's breaking away from the primary cancer; 3) the metastatic cell's entry in the blood vessels or lymphatic channels; 4) the metastatic cell's circulation; 5) its exist from the blood vessels or lymphatic channels by means of diapedesis and 6) the attachment of the metastatic cells to a new place.

Among the processes in which the normal eukaryotic somatic cells-built programs participate during the body's vital activity, the following should be mentioned: mitosis, diferentiation, interphase, phagocytosis, endomitosis, apoptosis, necrobiosis, adhesion, and, certainly fusing. When speaking about biological essence of fusing, its possibility to create polyploidy in somatic cells (like endomitosis) that intensifies resistance of respective organ to negative environmental factors deserves mentioning. Regrettably, this necessary on the face of it for the organism process is associated with the risks of malignant transformation of the fusion-developed binuclear and polyploid cells.

As a result of karyogamy, i.e., after synchronous mitosis or simple mechanical assembly of nuclei heterokaryons (or homokaryons), mononuclear hybrid precancerous cells develops, with tetraploid set of chromosomes on initial stage of hybridization. Received as a result of somatic hybridization, the hybrid synkaryon is an precancerous cell, which exists in macro organism indefinitely for a long time. On the promotion stage, after the influence of perfect carcinogens or promoters on tissue, where precancerous cells pre-exist, in these cells, the chromosomal aberrations of different types and genes amplifications may arise. From the chromosomal aberrations, the most dangerous in carcinogenic respect are nonbalanced translocations, and also duplications, expressed in "complementation" of chromosomes' identical sites, having the same function. This event usually leads of genes' amplification, in consequence of which expression of genes (oncogenes), responsible for the control under the cellular proliferation, ultimately may originate. At the initiated stage of its formation, precancerous synkaryons evidently possess tetraploid or hypotetraploid set of chromosomes. Further, in the process of tumor progression after the segregation of some chromosomes, tumorous cells with aneuploid or even hyperdiploid set of chromosomes may arise. After this, tumorous cells with extreme polymorphism of karyotype and new abilities arise.

Notwithstanding the fact that a tumor substrate originates initially from one synkaryon, or despite its clonal character, in most cases, the tumorous cells of highly morphologic and cytogenetic polymorphism originate. Cellular subpopulations are constantly formed in the tumor focus without any obvious regularity and can coexist in the phenotypically and genotypically distinguished cells. Thus, malignant tumors have clonal origin and on initial stage consist of genetically identical cells. In the future, cellular substrate of tumors develops continuously and alters genetic properties. Karyogamic theory explains these facts by spontaneous somatic hybridization between tumorous cells, or tumorous and precancerous cells, or between tumorous and normal cells of tumor substrate.

At first site, the drawback of karyogamic theory is the existence of malignant neoplasms with diploid set of chromosomes on tumorous cells [14]. However, it is necessary to emphasize that diploid set of chromosomes in tumorous cells does not signify absence of process of somatic hybridization in these rare cases. In cancer cells, one part of 46 chromosomes (in case of human) maybe from one initial cell, but the other part of chromosomes may represent the second parent (initial) cell (pseudodiploid clone); for instance, 20+26. The above-mentioned quantity of chromosomes (46) is undoubtedly one of the most balanced for cancer cells.

It is interesting in this respect that in some malignant tumors there are marked near-diploid or hyperhaploid chromosome modes. A near-haploid chromosome number of 29 to 30 was found in a melanoma and in case of metastatic melanoma characterized by a hypohaploid chromosome number of 24 [15]. Kovacs and his co-authors (1988) communicated about 70 cases of renal cell carcinomas, which usually showed near-diploid chromosomal modes [16]. In our opinion, these near-haploid and near-diploid chromosomal modes are result of tumorous cells chromosomes' selective segregation during carcinogenesis.

Thus, genetic abnormalities could cause by plasmalemma aberrations by affecting integral, peripheral or amphitropic membrane proteins.

From the view of kariogamic theory of carcinogenesis we are trying to answer one of the most complex questions in oncology: are the chromosomal aberrations the cause or the consequence of the cancerous growth? We hypothesize that during initiation (formation of precancerous cells) chromosomal aberrations (quantitative aberrations) are on the third place after the perforations of the plasma membrane and fusogeny (formation of dikaryons and then synkaryons). During promotion stagechromosomal aberrations (first of all structural aberrations) are on the first place before the gene amplification. In the case of progression (formation of cancerous cells with a new genotypes and phenotypes) the sequence should be the same as for the initiation (perforations, fusogeny and after that _ chromosomal quantitative aberrations). So the role of chromosomal aberrations differs at the different stages of carcinogenesis, but there are no doubts about their causative connections: at the stages of initiation and progression chromosomal aberrations are among the main causative factors (after the plasmatic membrane perforations and fusogeny), while at the stage of promotion, the main causative factor is the structural chromosomal aberrations.

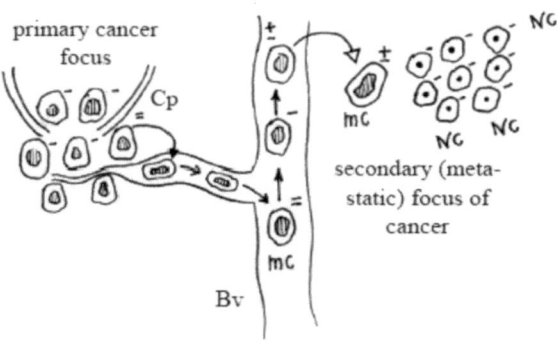

Fig. 3. Metastasis
Abbreviations: Bv – blood vessel; Cp – capillary;
Nc – normal cell; Mc – metastatic cell;
↘ - Penetration; ↝ - diapedesis;
- - negative charge; ± - neutral charge;
= - high negative charge.

CONCLUSION

During the perforation of the plasma membrane, induced by different carcinogenic agents, the total charge of this organoid changes and cells develop the ability to come closer to each other, which frequently, especially upon coincidence of the perforated parts, will probably be the prerequisite to a fusion process. In the process of promotion, the mechanism of malignant transformation probably has the molecular and subcellular conditions. Any combinations of cancer cell with other differentiated and nondifferentiated normal somatic cells are possible. New cellular subpopulations are constantly formed in tumors without any obvious regularity. Cancer cells have a variable membrane potential on their surface, which depends on the intensity of their metabolism and environmental hydrogen index. We suggest that the processes of invasion and metastasis can be ascribed to the presence of exactly this variable electric charge in a cancer cells. In contrast to metastasis, invasion process should take place only if cancer cells have a low negative, neutral or positive charge.

REFERENCES

1. Hallion, L. Le probleme du cancer et la biologie generale. *Press Med. Par.* 1907; XV:601-603.
2. Gogichadze, GK; Gogichadze, TG. *Karyogamic theory of cancer cell formation from the view of the XXI century.* Nova Biomedical Books, New York. 2010.
3. Gogichadze, GK; Gogichadze, TG. *Somatic hybridization, as a primary reason of malignization.* Lambert Academic Publisher, Saarbruken. 2013.
4. Gogichadze, GK; Gogichadze, TG; Kamkamidze, GK. Presumably common trigger mechanism of action of diametrically different carcinogens on target cells. *Cancer and Oncology Research.* 2013; 1(2):65-68.
5. Gogichadze, GK; Misabishvili, EV; Gogichadze, TG. Tumor cells formation by normal somatuic cells fusing and cancer prevention prospects. *Medical Hupotheses.* 2006; 66:133-136.
6. Meloni, G; Proia, A; Guerrisi, V. et al. Acute myeloid leukemia and lung cancer occurring in a chronic lymphocytic leukemia patient treated with fludarabine and autologous peripheral blood stem-cell transplantation. *Ann. Oncol.* 2000; 11:1493-1495.
7. Bea, S; Ribas, M; Hernandes, JM. et al. Increased number of chromosomal imbalances and DNA amplification on mantle cell lymphomas. *Ann. Oncol.* 1999; 10:101.
8. Heerema, NA; Nachman, JB; Sather, HN. et al. Hypodiploidy with less then 45 chromosomes confers adverse risk in childhood acute lymphoblastic leukemia: a report from the children's cancer group. *Blood.* 1999; 94:4036-4045.
9. Vanasse, GJ; Concannon, P; Willeford, DM. Review: regulated genomic instability and neoplasia in the lymphoid lineage. *Blood.* 1999, 94:3997-4010.
10. Sturm, SA; Strauss, PG; Adolph, S. et al. Amplification and rearrangment of C-myc in radiation-induced murine osteosarcomas. *Cancer Res.* 1990, 50:4146-4153.
11. Lonn, U; Lonn, S; Nylen, U. et al. Amplification of oncogenes in mammary carcinoma shown by fine-needle biopsy. *Cancer.* 1991; 67:1396-1400.
12. De Baetselier, P. *Neoplastic progression by somatic cell fusion.* Influence Tumor Dev. Host._ Dodrecht, etc. 1989.
13. Gogichadze, G; Gogichadze,T; Kamkamidze,G. Possible effect of variable membrane potential of a cancer cell on different carcinogenic processes. *Georgian Medical News.* 2014, 9 (234) :116-120.
14. Walker, J; Quirke, P. Biology and genetics of colorectal cancer. *Eur. J. Cancer.* 2001; 37:163-172.
15. Atkin, NB; Baker, MC. A metastatic malignant melanoma with 24 chromosomes. *Hum. Genet.* 1981; 58:217-219.
16. Kovacs, G; Soudah, B; Hoene, E. Binucleated cells in a human renal cell carcinoma with 34 chromosomes. *Cancer Genet. Cytogenet.* 1988; 31 : 211-215.

SUMMARY

The final part of this monograph is divided into 4 sections: 1) the quintessence of the provided data, where the essence of the karyogamic (two synkaryons) theory of carcinogenesis is given and the main theses of this theory are substantiated; 2) the main data in evidence of the karyogamic theory, both experimental and clinical, as well as logical proof; 3) the currently available cancer prevention and control means; and 4) the cancer therapy prospects.

1.Regrettably, our knowledge of the mechanisms of carcinogenesis is rather limited and insufficient. In other words, currently present is the lack of true information about initiation, promotion, progression (invasion, metastasis) and the critical molecular and sub-cellular phenomena taking place at these stages.

According to the Nowell's conception, tumors being clonal by origin, initially (at the first stages of development) consist of genetically identical cells, In the future, cellular substrate of tumors develops continuously and alters genetic properties. As a result, the highly stable cells that are suited to any unfavorable environmental conditions arise.

At the current stage of carcinogenesis development a question arises, whether malignization belongs to one of the most spread process (namely to fusogeny), which occurs in the body on a daily basis. Especially as the latest research evidences, this fusogenic activity is genetically programmed in somatic (and even non-somatic) cells.

Currently the most popular and reasoned theories and hypotheses of carcinogenesis are the theory of oncogenes, virus-genetic, immunological and polyetiological theories. Some theories of carcinogenesis are limited within the frames of etiology (for example, polyetiological theory), while the others – within the frames of pathogenesis (mutation and chromosomal theories). Only in rare cases they concern etiology, as well as pathogenetic aspects of the malignant growth simultaneously (for instance, virus-genetic theory of carcinogenesis).

In our opinion, the majority of the theses of the apologists of the virus-genetic theory do not agree with the major postulates of the karyogamic theory. For example, according to the apologists of the virus-genetic theory (and, possible, of other theories of carcinogenesis):

1. "It is hard to imagine that any effects on the cell surface can change its genome". Whereas one of the principal posulates of the karyogamic theory denote the changes occurred in the plasmalemma, which in the end finds reflection in the genome.

2. "It is hard to imagine that the changes induced by ionizing radiation, chemical carcinogens and viruses could be adequate". Answer on this thesis see on chapter 8 of this monograph.

3. "They (apologists of the virus-genetic theory. G.G.) stick to the hypothesis, under which only one cause of tumor formation – virus exists. As for pathogenesis, it is complex and the realization of pathogenicity of an etiological agent is conditioned by many causes". In other words, according to the virus-genetic theory, cancer is a monoetiological and concurrently polypathogenic process, which diametrically opposes the karyogamic theory positions.

4. "Spumaviruses are devoid of oncogenic properties . . . but induce the formation of syncytiums or fusion of cells". According to the karyogamic theory, if spumavirus (or any other agens) possesses fusogenic properties, it should also have the carcinogenic potential.

Only 2 postulates of the virus-genetic theory are acceptable for the karyogamic theory are acceptable for the karyogamic theory: 1) "The changes taken place in the target cell genome are of hereditary nature" and 2)" . . . the virus only initiates a tumor process and does not participate in the further stages of carcinogenesis. Thus, the virus is the initiator". This postulates are fully acceptable in terms of the karyogamic theory positions as well. The said fact, or the virus role in the initiation process, denotes the peculiarities of the oncological disease and its differences from diseases of other type, including an infectious diseases. The other differing from the latter circumstance consists in the fact that the clinical picture of cancer is defined not by the virus itself but by the growth (proliferation) of cancer cells thereby.

For the first time the karyogamic theory of carcinogenesis was suggested by French scientist Lui Hallion (1862-1940) at 1907. It is exactly in honor of Luis Hallion that we have called the theory proposed by us the "karyogamic theory" and only seldom use the "two synkaryons" or "hybridization" theories.

Beginning from 1970, interest to karyogamic theory of carcinogenesis has gradually but slowly increased (Mekler, Elkort, Klein, Gogichadze, Qiann, Duelli). Tisseuil, Higgins and Fekete suggested that origination of first malignant cell may be the result of fertilization or parthenogenesis between somatic cells or somatic cells and sperm cells.

As it is well-known, carcinogenesis consists of 3 stages: initiation, promotion and progression. The stage I of carcinogenesis – initiation attracts special attention because of 3 reasons: 1) initiation is the principal, initial, trigger stage of the carcinogenesis process; 2) according to the karyogamic theory, any agent or effect that induces fusogeny and somatic hybridization should be considered as a potential carcinogen; and 3) the initiation stage encompasses several sequential processes (steps) to be necessarily taken into account by the researcher working in experimental carcinogenesis.

At the first stage of carcinogenesis, i.e., at the stage of initiation, two (or more) normal somatic cells of one organ or tissue at some favorable conditions may create dikaryons (hetero- or homokaryons), but in some cases nonviable polykaryocytes. Presumably, during the perforation of plasmalemma induced by different carcinogenic and non-carcinogenic agents and factors, the total negative electric charge of this organoid changes, and the cells acquire the capacity of closely approaching (adhesion), which frequently, especially upon coincidence of the perforated parts, may serve as a prerequisite to fusion process.

The effects of physical, chemical, and biological carcinogenic agents on cells are probably adequate. They trigger the fusion of cells as a result of perforations of cytoplasmic membranes, i.e., the formation of pores in the plasmalemma, which induces the alteration of summary superficial charge on the cell surface. Because of this, cells acquire the ability to approach each other, which in many cases may be a premise for the fusion process. Thus, the initial target of carcinogenic agents is the cell plasma membrane, but not the genetic apparatus of somatic cells.

Thus, the immediate cause of the formation of a precancerous cell at the initiation stage is somatic hybridization, which itself consists of a whole number of sequential processes: a) production in plasma membranes of perforations of definite size/number under the effect of the so-called pore-producing agents (some viruses, toxins, particularly membranotoxins, various kinds of radiation, chemical carcinogens, etc.); b) loss of electron and proton homeostasis and reduction of the summary charge on the plasma membranes as a result of their subsequent perforations; c) approach and further contact of neighbour cells; d) adhesion of cells; e) fusogeny (upon coincidence of the perforated sites of plasmalemma; fusion of cytoplasmas of 2 neighbour cells with the formation of a dikaryon; f) karyogamy (fusion of 2 nuclei of the dikaryon in one structure) and g) formation of a precancerous cell (uninucleate, hybrid synkaryon).

At the initiated stage of its formation, precancerous synkaryons evidently possess tetraploid or hypotetraploid sets of chromosomes. Fusion process immediately doubles the number of chromosomes, thereby decreasing the chances that the loss of some chromosomes will kill the hybrid cell.

Further, in the process of tumor promotion after the segregation of some chromosomes, there may arise cancer cells with aneuploid or even hypodiploid set of chromosomes. In extremely rare cases, tumor cells possess even diploid, hypodiploid or even hyperhaploid sets of chromosomes. In this process of carcinogenesis, segregation of some chromosomes in the tumor synkaryon, and also involvement last cells by means of fusion of considerably amount of other tumor cells and normal cells of different types and maturity take place. After this, cancer cells with extreme polymorphism of the karyotype and new abilities arise.

A wide variety of agents (e.g. chemical carcinogens, radiations, some viruses, toxins, low pH, et al.) act at the level of the plasma membrane to cause structural alterations (perforations), which deteriorates the summary negative charge of the surface of somatic cells [1-3]. As a result, the neighbour cells will be enabled to approach one another, enter into contact and subject to adhesion and coincidence of the perforated sections of plasma membranes, a dikaryon – homo- or heterokaryons may be produced [4,5].

On the basis of an analysis of the above-mentioned data (chapters 1-10), it can be concluded that any agent or effect capable of inducing perforations in the plasma membranes of the target cells may be considered as a potential carcinogen. Such agents and effects include: some viruses, radiation of different kinds, chemical substances (carcinogens, pesticides, etc.), industrial, bio- and bacterial toxins, food substances (fatty acids, carbohydrates, etc.) and so on. The same perforating effect on the plasma membranes of the target cells can render both humoral (antibodies) and cellular immunity reagents (e.g., through immune cytolysis during allotransplantations), etc.

In our opinion, the common mechanism of action of diametrically different carcinogens on target-cells is the destruction of the plasmatic membrane (induction of the different size perforations) and consequently development of fusogeny – fusion of somatic cells, which is characteristics for any somatic cells and finally development of karyogamy (or reunion of nuclei). Thus, by karyogamic theory of carcinogenesis, initiated agents in the first instance interact with the cells plasma membranes, inducing their disintegration (perforations), fusion process and then cells' somatic hybridization (i.e. quantitative aberrations of chromosomes). As a result of this tetraploid (in some cases hypotetraploid) cells are formed.

It could be concluded that physical, chemical, and biological carcinogens lead to similar result: to induction of cells malignization by means of plasma membranes defects that produce abnormal electron and proton efflux, i.e. loss of electron and proton homeostasis. This defect (in other words, perforations) can be induced by a wide variety of agents, such as some viruses, chemical carcinogens, irradiations, toxins and so on. After perforations begins process of fusogeny and somatic hybridization. The formed as a result of this process heterokaryons, homokaryons and synkaryons are to be considered as basis of malignant growth.

As regards the carcinogenic action of some viruses, according to the karyogamic theory (the theory of hybridization, "two synkaryons") of carcinogenesis, the primary target of the virus (and other carcinogenic agents) is not the genetic apparatus of the somatic cell but the determinants localized on the cell's plasma membranes. It could be concluded that physical, chemical, and biological carcinogens lead to similar results: to induction of cells malignization by means of perforation of plasma membranes, adhesion, fusion and then somatic hybridization.

As it seems, the intensity of virus infections and the virulent properties of the virus itself acquire a decisive importance in the development of all types of pathologies (e.g., infections, tumors, etc.), to be followed by the formation of pores of different volume and amount in the process of the target cell plasma membrane perforations in the process of penetration or budding.

Some bacterial membranotoxins (and other biotoxins) of different tropism are capable, as a result of disintegrations (perforations) of the plasma membrane of the target cell of various degrees, of inducing both infectious processes as well as the formation of first precancerous and then cancer cells.

In hemolytic anemias of different genesis side by side with hemolysis, process of somatic cells fusion may take place. For instance, after bite of snake with hemolytic action of venom (*Vipera lebetina, Vipera Russellii*, etc.) together with massive destruction of erythrocytes (hemolysis), there may be induced fusion process of other cellular types with more rigid plasma membranes (for instance, leucocytes of different maturity, and probably of cells of other type), with possible development of a true malignant cell. Approximately similar action one may expect from fungus toxins (*Aspergillus flavus, Penicillium islandicum* and *Aspergillus ochraceus,* etc.). For instance, the toxin of *Aspergillus flavus* – aflatoxin together with heavy toxic action induces malignant tumors of liver.

Some dietary fats and carbohydrates too may induce perforations or modifications of somatic cell's plasma membranes in several conditions. This fact plays a definite role in the process of fusion and in arising of the tumor cells.

Distilled water and saline has capacity for destroying somatic cell's plasma membranes. Perforation of this organoid is a reason of cellular membranes fusion. Daily injection of distilled water and saline into laboratory animals may induce perforations of plasma membranes, which assist their approach and following fusion.

In case of allotransplantation, during the perforation of cellular membranes induced by antibodies or T-killers, the total charge of plasma membranes changes, and the cells acquire the capability of closely approaching (adhesion), which frequently, especially upon coincidence of the perforated parts, may serve as a prerequisite to fusion. Thus, a situation may occur in the recipient, when on attack of a macrophage or cytotoxic T-lymphocyte (killer) on a normal cell partner cells are not perished but fuse and form somatic hybrids.

For example, it has been found that definite concentrations of alcohol act on the lipid-like substances of the cellular membranes, causing perforations in this organoid, by which its permeability is dramatically affected. By means of an epidemiologic analysis it was found that whisky, calvados, vodka and other strong drinks contribute frequently to the development of cancer in the human body. For most oncologists (in any case for those who do not share the karyogamic theory of carcinogenesis) it is hard to imagine through which way and by which mechanism definite concentrations of alcohol can contribute to the development of cancer. As for the followers of the karyogamic theory, they believe that as alcohol can induce the production of perforations of definite size and quantity in the plasma membranes, then subject to coincidence of the perforated sections in the plasma membranes of two neighbor cells, first a dikaryon (binucleate) and then a precancerous cell can be formed, with the hardest resultant consequences.

In addition to a specific effect of different pathogens (viruses, bacterial toxins, biotoxins of other types) on the plasma membrane of the target cells, being reflected in the formation of perforations of different number (Pq – perforation quantities) and volume, size (Pv – perforation volum), approximately the same effect can be characteristic of the so-called immune (both cell-immune and humor-immune) cytolysis. In the case of both cell-immune and humor-immune cytolysis, the perforations formed on the target cell plasmalemma may become a direct cause of various cytopathogenic and clinical manifestations. Depending on the number and size of the pores, different, often diametrically opposite pathologies (e.g., infections and cancer) can develop (see Chapter 2 about viruses for details).

Thus, based on the positions of the karyogamic theory (hybridization, "two synkaryons" theory), it is possible to establish sequences of malignant transformation of a normal cell according to stages. A special emphasis should be made on the carcinogenesis **initiation** stage. As has already been mentioned, the said stage (initiation) consists of the following 4 steps:

Step I of initiation _ perforations of the plasma membranes of the target cells. As has been established, any carcinogenic or non-carcinogenic agent (virus, radiation, toxin, carbohydrate, fatty acid, low pH, distilled water, etc.) has a common mechanism of action on the target cell: they all induce perforations or the production of pores (holes) in the plasmalemma of the target cells. Much importance is given to the pores' quantity (Pq) and volume (Pv). This phenomenon may become a prerequisite for reduction of the summary negative charge on the cell's surface and approach of the cells. As it seems, the degree of perfo- rations (pores' quantity- Pq and pores' volume - Pv) should be of decisive importance in the realization of any clinical state (infection, tumor process, teratogeny, etc.). It should be mentioned here that in the case of perforations of different degrees of the plasma membrane of the target cells, varying clinical manifestations may take place:

a. In the case of development of big size pores (approximately 8-10 to 100 nm) or upon their massive formation _ rapid repair of the plasma membrane by the cell becomes impossible and the cell undergoes irreversible changes – destruction (cytolysis), e.g., because of direct cytotoxic effect of the virus, radiation, toxin. The clinical manifestation of the above may be the development of any infectious process;

b. In the case of development of lesser size pores _ the transformation of the target cells into giant, nonviable polykaryocytes. Three- and more nucleate (rarely 500-nucleate) polykaryocytes may be formed. The latter represent the so-called genetic impasse, for they fail to enter the S-phase of the cell cycle, subsequent mitosis and tend to be soon destroyed. The clinical manifestation of the above may be an infectious process, immune deficiency, teratogeny, but in no case a malignant process;

c. In the case of development of still lesser size pores _ the formation of a precancerous (immortalized, initiated) cell, the direct cause of which might be a reduction of the summary negative charge on the surface of the plasma membrane of 2 neighbour normal somatic cells.

Step II of initiation _ approach of two normal somatic cells, their contact and follow-up adhesion.

Step III of initiation _ fusogeny. In case of coincidence of the perforated parts of the plasmalemma of 2 neighbour somatic cells, a binucleate cell of high oncogenic potency – dikaryon (hetero- or homo- karyon) may be formed.

Step IV of initiation _ karyogamy and then tetraploidy (at the early stage of a precancerous cell formation). As a result of synchronous mitosis of the dikaryons, a uninucleate hybrid cell – synkaryon, with a tetraploid set of chromosomes, may be formed at the early stage of development of precancerous cell. Possibly, in addition to the synchronous mitosis (when a division spindle is formed), a mechanical fusion of interphase nuclei may also occur. The high synchronization degree and normal development of mitosis occurs irrespective of the interphase period in which the fused nuclei of somatic cells are. At this stage, the cell may be called a precancerous (initiated, immortalized) cell. Thereafter, the phenomenon of chromosomes' segregation will take place.

For tumor **promotion** (i.e. formation of a tumor synkaryon) the necessary precondition is active proliferation, i.e. hyperplasia of the corresponding tissue. Under the effect of complete carcinogens, promoters, non-specific influences or some extreme situations, a precancerous synkaryon can transform into a tumor synkaryon. The pre-existence in the corresponding tissue and organs of precancerous cells has been described elsewhere. The carcinogenic effect of promoters is due to their action on latent precancerous cells in target organs. The mechanism of malignant transformation of the precancerous cell into a tumor cell probably has the molecular and sub-cellular foundation. In terms of oncology, particular dangerous are: chromosomal translocations (especially of non-balanced type), duplications, deletion and gene amplifications. This may lead to the development of aneuploidy and arising of true cancerous cell.

Carcinogenesis stage III _ **progression** should seemingly be initiated in two processes – invasive and metastatic. The first, or the invasive process, is developed by involvement of new, intact cells and tissues into carcinogenesis, where a great role should be again given to somatic hybridization. At this time, malignant cells of a new type are being formed. As it is well-known, the genotypic and phenotypic instability is the primary manifestation in cancer. In the second manifestation of the progression (metastasis), or the arising of secondary tumor loci, the key role should be given to the variable electric potential of the cancer cells (see Chapter 10 for details).

2. In this section of the "Summary" we shall attempt to briefly corroborate the validity of the karyogamic theory of carcinogenesis. Is not this theory the key that, to say it artistically, opens almost all the closed up to now secret doors to oncology? In other words, does this theory answer some currently unanswered questions of carcinogenesis (and not only carcinogenesis)? For example, how the dual, diametrically opposite pathological processes of some viruses (or toxins) can be understood? (Chapter 2); or how can the common genesis of infectious and oncogenic viruses be conceived? (Sub-chapter 2b); in what is expressed the common mechanism of different, diametrically opposed nature of carcinogenic (and of non-carcinogenic) agents and factors (chemical substances, radiation, viruses, low pH, Biotoxins, etc.) on the target cells? (Chapters 3, 4, 8); what is the essence of the molecular and genetic aspects of carcinogenesis? (Chapter 10), etc. We believe that these questions have been rather convincingly answered from the standpoint of the karyogamic theory of carcinogenesis.

Moreover, another important circumstances should be underlined: the hybridoma production scheme and the carcinogenesis initiation scheme presented by us are very similar, may even be identical, although differing by the type of cells involved in the process: in the first case, a hybrid synkaryon (hybridoma) produced as a result of fusion and karyogamy of B-lymphocyte and myeloma cell and separates mononuclear antibodies; as for the second case, the synkaryon produced as a result of fusion of 2 normal somatic cells represents a precancerous (initiated, immortalized) cell. Simply, in the second case, although infrequently, the development of a dramatic for the macro organism situation is still expected: transformation of a precancerous cell into a tumorous cell at the stage of promotion. Thus, one of the evidence of the scheme provided by us (at least including the stage of initiation) is the fact of production of hybridomas, which has been repeatedly established by different leading scientists, namely by Köhler and Milstein [6] and others.

It is also of interest to mention the fact that for producing hybridomas the diametrically opposite agents and factors are used: Sendai virus, polyethylene glycol, membrane-active substances _ lysolecithin, polyarginine, as well as calcium ions, low pH, sucrose, glyceryl monooleate, antibodies, electric fields, radiation of different nature and laser impulses. All of them induce a rupture of the plasmalemma of individual parts of somatic cells (B-lymphocytes and myeloma cells), the negative charge deterioration, first approach of cells, then contact, fusogeny (with the production of binucleate cells) and somatic hybridization, or the unification of cellular nuclei and formation of hybridomas. It is very probable that mechanism of cells' fusion in tissue culture and *in vivo* is adequate for different agents and factors. The agents and factors of about the same nature induce the malignant transformation of a normal cell.

Another evidence of the initiation scheme validity is a short-term test for fusogeny of different carcinogenic agents, factors and effects. As we believe, the above-mentioned substances and factors that induce the cells' fusion are potentially oncogenic ones. The positive fusogenic effect (i.e., appearance of two- and polynuclear hetero- and homokaryons) of all the known carcinogens with negative controls can confirm the existence exactly this mechanism in malignization and also allows the use this method for the determination of carcinogenicity of certain chemical substances and other dubious factors in an oncogenic respect [7,8]. It is necessary to emphasize that approximately such results were received relatively later by Baldwin and Lucy [9].

Based on the above, the validity of the carcinogenesis initiation scheme proposed by us does not give rise to any doubts.

It is generally agreed that karyogamic (hybridization, two synkaryons) theory, is hardly subject to experimental corroboration. True, to all appearance no proper experimental material in evidence of this theory has been produced up to now. In our opinion, such material is available, namely the 1987 data provided by Behringer and his co-authors [10] concerning the Friend's virus (with the use of allophenic animals) and the duplication of the same data by us almost 20 years later, although using another virus, namely the Moloney virus and the linear mice responsive to this virus [11], is the direct experimental proof of the karyogamic theory. It should also be noted that much earlier than Behringer, Elkort in 1972 and then Mekler in 1976 proved experimentally the hybridization theory of malignant cell formation [12,13], but, unfortunately, they obtained rather unconvincing data, which they themselves (for example, Mekler) acknowledged.

It would be expedient for proving the hybridization of somatic cells later to use the so-called microfilming technique in the cell culture.

As regards the promotion stage, further observations, experimental analysis, logical proofs, etc, will be required in order to finally corroborate the idea on this stage proposed by us.

3. We understand it well that however much we write or speak about the essence of a malignant process, the first question which any reader will ask would be the following: Well, we already know what the malignant cell is, what is its essence, but have we managed to advance a bit in its treatment? Has the contemporary science managed to find a potent anticancer remedy? A child and an adult, an educated and an uneducated person, a doctor and a lawyer, etc., all of them can bring up such embarrassing and unanswerable questions at the current stage of medicine development. Do we have the right and intelligible answer to this question? Unfortunately, not! And yet, in spite of everything, we shall still try to be more optimistic and to answer it within the limits of the possible!

We acknowledge that the theory proposed by us is rather pessimistic and in spite of a new vision of the essence of cancer stated therein, it does not create the elevated and optimistic mood neither in the reader not in us, and still…

If the scheme proposed by us contains any rational kernel, we should try to identify the weakest, relatively easily surmountable point (stage, step) on the way a genuine cancer cell is formed and try to act correspondingly. To our mind, the weakest point is the initiation stage of carcinogenesis and its constituent initial steps: beginning with the plasma membrane perforation and ending with fusogeny.

In our opinion, new strategies to reduce significantly the risk of cancer should be developed.

The effect of cell surface will finally find its reflection in the genome. In other words, cancer is the genome's disorder and it is quite natural to expect progress in the treatment of such a patient only if the process determining and regulating the normal and parthological functioning of the cell genome are studied.

For preventing this fatal disease, the inhibition of the process of approaching and further adhesion of normal somatic cells would suffice. The expected outcome would be the creation on the body of the conditions when somatic cells are incapable of close contacts with each other (not injurious for macro organism). This will completely exclude the fusion of cells and then nuclei (karyogamy) and reduce thus to a minimum, the possibility of cancer cell development. In technical terms, this is a considerably easily performed process as against the manipulation in the genome at the molecular level (for dehybridization) or the repression of the genes being responsible for malignant transformation.

To achieve the set objective, it would be ideal to use the cell plasma membranes' stabilizing substances (to avoid perforations of this organoid), or the low-molecular disaggregants (for inhibition of narrow contacts and following cells' adhesion). These substances might be administered to the person permanently, in the course of life, in small, harmless doses (for example with drinking water and food). The expected outcome would be the creation in the macro organism of the conditions when somatic cells are incapable of close contacts with each other. This will almost completely exclude the fusion of somatic cells and then nuclei and reduce, to a minimum the possibility of cancer cell development.

The method suggested by us is not certainly absolute, but it, we believe, can significantly reduce (but not eradicate) the development of malignant tumors in the human body. Especially since, as has already been mentioned, a cancer cell may also be formed spontaneously. It should also be said that the implementation of this idea requires much efforts and, most important, time, while mankind awaits something momentary, some panacea, which at the present stage of development we believe is an unattainable dream.

As regards repair process of perforated sites of plasma membrane, it's possible to used ceramide and other substances.

4. The "magic bullet" of the great scientist Paul Ehrlich, which had proved rather effective in treating infectious diseases, failed to justify hopes in the case of cancer cure. Regrettably, polychemotherapy, as well as radiation therapy, tends to damage both the malignant and healthy cells, and this fact should not be overlooked. Seemingly, a principally different way, different approach should be looked for in this direction.

Since man lives in the unsterile environment and is surrounded by different kinds of bacteria and viruses, as well as carcinogenic substances and factors, his complete isolation from the initiators and carcinogens inducing a tumor process is very hard (even impossible).

It is a great pity that all the methods existing up-to-date to defeat the cancer (be it chemotherapy, surgery, immunotherapy, X-ray therapy and others) turned out to be not so effective. So, the research of the data still continues.

Hence, the lack of vital capacity of fused polykaryocytes and the fact that they perish briefly, gives us the right to make a supposition, that if it is possible to transfer tumor cells synchronously in the stage of polykaryocytes, then it is possible to dissociate the tumor substrate and to diminish the whole mass of tumor and even its resolution [14]. Moreover, it is already stated that the tumor cells, in comparison with the normal ones, are more sensitive to the influence of different fusogenic agents or they more easy transform to the stage of nonviable polykaryocytes. It should be mentioned here that the idea of the transformation of the cancer substrate into unviable polykaryocytes for cancer treatment proposed by us [14], later, in 2002 was reiterated by Peng and his co-authors [15] on another model.

How can we achieve the transformation of tumor cells to the stage of nonviable polykaryocytes? It would be ideal to find out such chemical substances, biological agents and so on, which alongside with the fusogenic qualities would have the ability of tropism to either tissue or organ. Carcinogenic substances, whose tropism to either tissue or organ is stated for a long time, reveal their fusogenic qualities very weakly [7,8]. It is not perspective to use Sendai virus in this concrete case, as its tropism is characteristic only for the mucous membranes. Although the viruses of fusogenic qualities can be used, which have tropism for either tissue or organ (e.g., cytomegaloviruses, other herpes viruses, hepatitis viruses, etc.). It should be mentioned here that the idea developed by us, can be found more efficient in the case of the so-called compact rather than diffuse tumors.

To our mind, it must be perspective to introduce in cancer organ (i.e., cancer itself) by means of echoscopy control 55-60% solution of polyethylene glycol with dimethylsulfoxide. We suppose that the origin of polykaryocytes will set in 1-2 hours, and in 48-55 hours their total destruction will begin, i.e., the dissociation and diminishment of cancer. The above-mentioned method is said to be paradoxical, as for the treatment of cancer are given the substances and agents, the certain doses of which induce dikaryons of high cancer potency.

REFERENCES

1. Arvinte, T; Cudd, A; Schulz, B. et al. Low-pH associated of proteins with the membranes of intact red blood cells. II. Studies of the mechanism. *Bioch. et Bioph. Acts.* 1989; 981:61-68.
2. Siroki, J; Cervenka J. Hybridization frequency of different mammalian cell types by electrofusion. *Gen.Physiol. Biophys.* 1990; 9:489-499.
3. Gogichadze, GK; Misabishvili, EV; Gogichadze TG. Tumor cells formation by normal somatic cells fusing and cancer prevention prospects. *Med. Hypotheses.* 2006; 66 :133-136.
4. Gogichadze, GK; Gogichadze, TG. *Karyogamic theory of cancer cell formation from the view of the XXI century.* Nova Biomedical Books, New York. 2010.
5. Gogichadze, GK. *Common characteristics of a cancer cell and logical corroborations of its hybrid essence.* Advances in Genetic Research. Ed. Kevin Urbano. 2011; 46:161-178.
6. Kohler, G; Milstein, C. Continuous cultures of fused cells secreting antibody of prodefined specificity. *Nature.* 1975; 256:495-497
7. Gogichadze, GK; Piriashvili, VA; Abesadze, AI. *The action of some chemical carcinogens on nuclear erythrocytes.* Bulletin of the Academy of Sciences of Georgia. 1991; 141:397-400.
8. Gogichadze, GK; Dolidze, TG., Beniashvili, D. et al. *Short-term bioassay for confirmation of carcinogenic properties in various chemical substances.* Int Conf. Int. Fed. Soc.of Toxicol. Pathologists "Current Methods for the Evaluation of Pathology in Toxicology", Nagoya, Japan, 1992, 32.

9. Baldwin, JM; Lucy JA. Chemically induces fusion of erythrocyte membranes. *Methods Enzymol.* 1993; 220:161-173.
10. Behringer, RR; LoCascio, NJ; Dewey, MJ. Erythroid cell fusion in the early phase of Friend virus leukemogenesis. *J.Natl. Cancer Inst.* 1987; 79:601-603.
11. Gogichadze, GK; Beniashvili, D; Gogichadze, T. Fusogenic Effects of Lymphoid Cells at Early Stages of Moloney Virus-Induced Lympholeukemia. *Experimental and Clinical Medicine.* 2008; 5:9-13.
12. Elkort, RJ; Handler, AH; Kobrick, S. et al. The relationship of somatic cell hybridization to carcinogenesis. *Europ. J. Cancer.* 1972; 8:259-261.
13. Mekler, LB; Artamonova, SI; Bodyagin, DA. et al. IV. Somatic hybridization and oncogenesis: induction of tumors in mice as a result of the injection of mixtures of cells of the homologous organs and their hybrids. *Ontogenesis.* 1976; 7:246-254.
14. Gogichadze, GK; Gedenidze, AV. A Paradoxical Idea of Cancer's Resolution. *Med. Hypotheses.* 2000; 55:300-301.
15. Peng, K-W; TenEyck, CJ; Galanis, E. et al. Intraperitoneal therapy of ovarian cancer using an engineered measles virus. *Cancer Res.* 2002; 62:4656-4662.